BASIC
FIRST AID MANUAL
GUIDE

Dr. Charlotte Roark

Copyright Page: © 2023 by Dr. Charlotte Roark

Disclaimer

The information provided in this book, authored by Dr. Charlotte Roark, is intended for educational purposes only. It is not a substitute for professional medical advice, diagnosis, or treatment. Always seek the advice of your physician or other qualified healthcare provider with any questions you may have regarding a medical condition. Never disregard professional medical advice or delay in seeking it because of something you have read in this book.

The author and publisher of this book make no representations or warranties with respect to the accuracy, applicability, fitness, or completeness of the contents of this book. They disclaim any warranties (expressed or implied), merchantability, or fitness for any particular purpose. The author and publisher shall in no event be held liable for any loss or other damages, including but not limited to special, incidental, consequential, or other damages.

TABLE OF CONTENT

INTRODUCTION

Emily was happy. It was a typical Saturday afternoon, and she was enjoying a leisurely stroll in the park with her younger sister, Sarah. The sun was shining, birds were chirping, and laughter filled the air as children played nearby.

As they walked, Sarah suddenly tripped over a tree root and fell hard onto the ground, crying out in pain. Emily rushed to her side and saw that Sarah was clutching her arm, tears streaming down her face. Emily's heart raced with panic as she assessed the situation. Sarah's arm was twisted at an unnatural angle, and she winced with every movement.

In that moment of crisis, Emily's mind flashed back to the lessons she had recently learned about first aid. Remembering the importance of stabilizing the injury, she quickly retrieved the book from her backpack and flipped to the section on fractures.

Emily followed the steps outlined in her course to design a makeshift splint using a nearby stick and a scarf. Drawing upon the knowledge she had gained from reading the manual, she carefully immobilized Sarah's arm, providing relief from the pain and preventing further damage.

As Sarah's cries subsided and she began to relax, Emily felt a sense of pride and gratitude wash over her. She had been able to spring into action with confidence and competence, ultimately saving her sister from further harm.

In "Basic First Aid Manual Guide," we've endeavored to equip you with the essential knowledge and skills needed to respond confidently and effectively in emergency situations. Whether you're faced with minor injuries, common illnesses, or life-threatening emergencies, this comprehensive guide provides clear, step-by-step instructions, accompanied by helpful illustrations, to empower you to take action when it matters most. From assembling a first aid kit to performing CPR and managing environmental hazards, each chapter is designed to arm you with the tools and know-how to provide immediate care and support to those in need. With "Basic First Aid Manual Guide" by your side, you can approach any emergency with preparedness, confidence, and the assurance that you have the skills to make a difference.

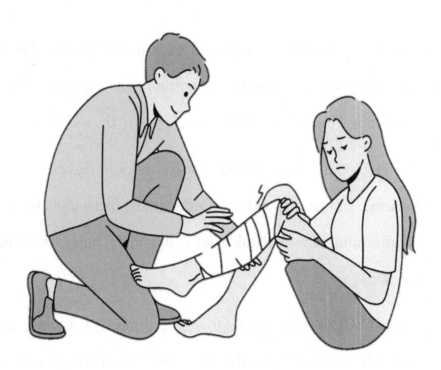

CHAPTER 1: FOUNDATIONAL KNOWLEDGE

Understanding the basic knowledge about first aid is crucial for effectively responding to emergencies. Foundational knowledge encompasses fundamental principles such as recognizing the signs of distress, assessing the severity of injuries, and knowing when to seek professional medical assistance. It involves grasping the basics of wound care, CPR, and the importance of maintaining a safe and sterile environment. By mastering these foundational concepts, individuals can become empowered to act swiftly and confidently in emergency situations, potentially saving lives and minimizing harm. In essence, foundational knowledge serves as the cornerstone upon which effective first aid practices are built, ensuring preparedness and readiness to respond when the need arises.

What Is First Aid?

First aid is the immediate medical care provided right at the scene of an injury or accident. It's the initial response that can make all the difference, often requiring minimal equipment or expertise to administer. Think of it as the crucial first step before professional medical help arrives. First aid can encompass a range of actions, from cleaning minor cuts and scrapes to soothing minor burns and applying bandages. It's about simple yet essential techniques like draining blisters, removing debris from the eyes, or even offering a comforting massage. In cases of heat stress, hydrating with fluids can also be part of the first aid repertoire. Ultimately, first aid is about being ready to lend a helping hand when someone needs it most, with basic but effective interventions that can truly save lives.

Your Role in First Aid Situations

In times of crisis, first aiders stand as pillars of support, trained to provide immediate care to those in need. Whether it's a workplace incident or a community event, these individuals are entrusted with the responsibility of safeguarding lives and ensuring the well-being of the injured or ill.

The Responsibilities of a First Aider

As a first aider, your primary duty revolves around delivering swift and effective medical assistance to those requiring urgent attention. From tending to minor wounds to stabilizing an unconscious individual, your actions can make a significant difference in the outcome of an emergency. Among your crucial tasks may include:

1. Safeguarding the airway of an unconscious person through careful positioning

2. Administering cardiopulmonary resuscitation (CPR) or utilizing automated external defibrillators (AEDs)

3. Applying appropriate pressure to control external bleeding

4. Providing support and care for injured limbs

Additional Roles of First Aiders

Beyond these core responsibilities, first aiders often find themselves fulfilling distinct roles tailored to their specific assignments and qualifications.

Workplace First Aider

In workplace settings, the presence of a trained first aider is indispensable. Responsible for attending to employees in the event of a health crisis, workplace first aiders play a crucial role in maintaining a safe and secure work environment. With regulations mandating employers to prioritize employee safety, the need for workplace first aiders, equipped with essential certifications and resources, is paramount.

Mental Health First Aider

Recognizing the importance of mental well-being, many workplaces now appoint mental health first aiders. These individuals provide vital support and guidance to colleagues facing mental health challenges, underscoring the significance of holistic wellness in the workplace.

Importance of First Aid

First aid is more than just a set of skills—it's a crucial aspect of emergency preparedness that can make a profound difference in saving lives and minimizing the impact of injuries and medical emergencies. Here are several key reasons why first aid is of paramount importance:

1. First Aid is a Lifesaving Skill: Recent statistics from The Guardian reveal a staggering truth: over 150,000 individuals suffer grave injuries or lose their lives annually due to a lack of first aid knowledge. In our modern age, where advancements in technology abound, this figure is a stark reminder of the critical importance of first aid training. Swift and proper administration of first aid can be the difference between life and death in emergencies, making it imperative for more individuals to acquire the necessary skills to respond effectively to accidents or medical crises. Heart attacks, choking incidents, and other life-threatening situations can be mitigated through prompt and informed care, highlighting the crucial role of first aid in saving lives.

2. Helps you stay prepared as accidents can strike anytime: The unpredictability of accidents and emergencies is an undeniable reality of life. In the United States alone, over six million people are involved in traffic accidents annually, making it the leading cause of death for individuals aged 1 to 54. Whether at home, work, or on the road, no one is immune to the possibility of encountering an unexpected crisis. Basic first aid skills such as CPR, wound disinfection, and bleeding control serve as invaluable tools that can make a significant difference in mitigating the impact of such emergencies. By equipping ourselves with these essential skills, we enhance our preparedness to respond effectively to unforeseen accidents or crises whenever and wherever they may occur.

3. Every Second Matters: In medical emergencies, the first few minutes are paramount. This critical window of time can make a substantial difference in preventing injuries from worsening until professional medical assistance arrives. Consider a scenario where a person experiences cardiac arrest: within just 3 to 4 minutes, the brain begins to suffer from oxygen deprivation. It is during these crucial minutes that swift action, such as administering CPR, can significantly improve the chances of survival and minimize long-term consequences. While calling for emergency services remains a priority, the ability to provide immediate first aid measures can play a pivotal role in stabilizing the patient's condition and increasing their likelihood of survival.

4. It is a catalyst for swift recovery: Beyond its life-saving potential, first aid also plays a vital role in expediting the recovery process for individuals affected by injuries. Failure to address injuries promptly can lead to severe complications such as hemorrhagic shock due to uncontrolled blood loss, resulting in prolonged recovery times and potentially permanent damage to tissues and organs. By promptly administering first aid measures to stop bleeding, stabilize injuries, and alleviate pain, individuals can facilitate a smoother and faster recovery process, reducing the risk of long-term complications and promoting overall well-being.

5. Alleviating Pain and Discomfort: Injuries and accidents often entail significant pain and discomfort for the affected individuals. While not life-threatening, these experiences can be distressing and overwhelming. One of the primary benefits of prompt first aid intervention is the ability to alleviate pain and discomfort, providing immediate relief and comfort to the injured party. By assessing and addressing pain promptly, trained individuals can ensure that the victim remains as comfortable as possible while awaiting further medical assistance, fostering a sense of reassurance and care during challenging times.

6. Empowerment Through Knowledge: Perhaps the most compelling reason to acquire first aid skills is the potential to save lives, including your own. In professions that entail inherent health risks or for individuals with pre-existing medical conditions, the ability to administer first aid can be a literal lifesaver. With proper training, individuals learn to remain calm and composed in emergency situations, enabling them to take decisive action and even guide others in life-threatening scenarios. This empowerment extends beyond immediate assistance, as individuals equipped with first aid knowledge can help raise awareness and promote a culture of safety within their communities.

7. Reducing the Burden of Medical Expenses: Effective first aid intervention not only saves lives but also contributes to reducing the burden of medical expenses. In cases where injuries are left unattended or exacerbated due to delayed intervention, the resulting complications often necessitate extensive medical treatment, leading to increased healthcare costs. Conversely, by promptly addressing injuries and preventing further deterioration through first aid measures, individuals can minimize the severity of injuries, mitigate complications, and ultimately reduce the associated medical expenses. This proactive approach to healthcare not only benefits individuals but also contributes to the overall efficiency of healthcare systems.

8. First Aid as a Valuable Skill Set: Beyond its life-saving potential and cost-saving benefits, first aid proficiency opens doors to a wide range of job opportunities across various industries. Many professions, including electricians, personal trainers, firefighters, social workers, and flight attendants, require individuals to possess adequate first aid training and certification. By acquiring and maintaining first aid credentials, individuals not only enhance their employability but also demonstrate their commitment to safety and well-being in the workplace. As employers increasingly prioritize health and safety standards, the demand for first aid-trained personnel continues to grow, making first aid proficiency a valuable asset in today's job market.

9. Cultivating Confidence and Security: Knowledge of first aid not only instills confidence in individuals but also fosters a sense of security within communities. By equipping individuals with the skills and knowledge to respond effectively to emergencies, first aid training promotes a culture of preparedness and resilience, empowering individuals to take proactive measures to safeguard themselves and those around them. Heightened awareness of potential risks and hazards enables individuals to assess situations accurately, take decisive action, and provide timely assistance when needed, thereby contributing to the overall safety and well-being of their communities.

10. Bridging the Gap: Despite the critical importance of first aid skills, research indicates that a significant portion of the population lacks adequate training in this essential area. According to studies conducted by the Red Cross, only a mere 5% of adults possess the skills and confidence to administer first aid in emergencies, with an alarming 71% admitting to feeling ill-prepared to respond if someone collapses in their presence. This knowledge deficit underscores the urgent need for widespread first aid education and training initiatives to bridge the gap and empower more individuals to respond effectively to emergencies. By undertaking first aid training, individuals not only acquire life-saving skills but also become catalysts for positive change within their communities, promoting safety, preparedness, and well-being for all.

Responding to Emergencies

Life is unpredictable, and emergencies can arise when we least expect them – whether we're at the supermarket, in our apartment lobby, or picking up the kids from school. Having the knowledge to respond effectively in such situations empowers us to act confidently and decisively.

Let's explore the Golden Rules of First Aid, encapsulated in the mnemonic **DRS ABCD**, which can be our guiding light in times of crisis.

D: Danger

As we approach the scene, our first instinct is to assess for any immediate dangers – from fire hazards to broken power lines. Our safety and that of others are paramount. If possible, we must remove the victim from harm's way while ensuring our own safety.

R: Response

Using the talk and touch method, we gauge the person's responsiveness. Are they conscious? If so, our priority is to make them comfortable and provide reassurance. We assess for any injuries and administer first aid as needed, promptly calling for professional assistance if required.

S: Send for Help

In an emergency, every second counts. We dial emergency services (such as 911) and provide precise details about our location and the nature of the situation. Clear communication ensures swift and effective response from emergency responders.

A: Airway

For conscious individuals, we ensure their airway is clear and that they're breathing normally. However, for the unconscious, we conduct a careful check for obstructions, clearing the airway if necessary using proper techniques.

B: Breathing

Normal breathing is a sign of life. We observe for chest movements, listen for breath sounds, and feel for airflow. If the person is breathing, we attend to any additional injuries before providing first aid.

C: CPR (Cardiopulmonary Resuscitation)

In the absence of breathing, we initiate CPR immediately. With proper technique – 30 compressions followed by 2 breaths – we strive to maintain circulation and oxygenation until professional help arrives. Utilizing a defibrillator if available can further improve the chances of survival.

D: Defibrillator

If accessible, a defibrillator can be a lifesaving tool in restoring normal heart rhythm. Continuing CPR while applying a defibrillator increases the likelihood of a positive outcome.

Remember: Familiarize yourself with defibrillator locations in places you frequent. Being prepared can make all the difference in saving a life.

Preventing Infection

Preventing the spread of infections during first aid procedures is paramount for both patient safety and the protection of first responders. Let's delve into strategies to mitigate cross infection risks, understanding its causes, associated risks, and essential equipment for infection control.

Understanding Cross Infection

Cross infection, or cross transmission, occurs when infections are transferred from one person to another. This can happen through direct contact, such as touching, or indirectly via contaminated surfaces or equipment. Respiratory infections like COVID-19 are often spread through droplets from coughing or sneezing, which can then be transferred by touching infected surfaces and subsequently touching the face.

Causes of Cross Infection: Infections can be caused by various microorganisms like bacteria, viruses, fungi, and parasites. In a first aid scenario, cross infection may arise from using contaminated dressings, coughing near the patient, or improper hand hygiene.

Risks and Complications: Cross infections can lead to severe health complications, including diarrhoea, pneumonia, sepsis, meningitis, organ failure, and even death. They can also impede the healing process for existing injuries or health conditions.

Prevention Measures: Utilizing personal protective equipment (PPE) like face masks and disposable gloves is crucial for preventing cross infection. Standard precautions include treating all body fluids as potentially infectious and ensuring safe disposal of needles and syringes.

Hand Hygiene: Proper hand hygiene is essential. Regular hand washing with soap and water or using alcohol-based hand rubs effectively removes germs from hands.

Disposable Gloves: Nitrile gloves reduce contamination risk when handling body fluids. They should be worn before and after handling patients and discarded if damaged or visibly soiled.

Face Masks: Disposable surgical masks offer protection against airborne viruses like COVID-19, influenza, and measles, when worn correctly.

Antiseptic Agents: Antiseptic wipes and liquids sterilize skin to prevent bacterial spread. They are crucial for wound care and skin preparation.

Sterile Dressings: Proper wound care reduces infection risks. When dressing wounds, ensure sterile gloves are used, and the dressing covers the wound entirely.

Safe Disposal of Clinical Waste: Contaminated items, including used wound dressings and gloves, must be disposed of safely to prevent infection spread.

First Aid Supplies for Infection Control

Having updated first aid supplies on hand is essential for delivering effective care during emergencies. Whether managing situations on the spot or awaiting further medical assistance, having the right equipment ensures safe and efficient first aid care.

Assessing Vital Signs

Vital signs, often referred to as life signs, are fundamental indicators that are assessed in a person to evaluate their current health status, stability, or any changes resulting from an illness or injury. These vital signs encompass various aspects such as coloration, body temperature, breathing rate, pulse, and level of consciousness, all of which play a crucial role in determining the individual's well-being. Regular monitoring of these vital signs is imperative during your interaction with the person in need. Particularly in situations where you may be providing assistance before professional medical help arrives, keeping a close eye on the casualty's vital signs becomes essential for timely and appropriate care.

When is it essential to evaluate vital signs in someone who's injured?

After conducting your Primary Survey, which involves checking the airway, breathing, and circulation, and contacting emergency services if necessary, it's crucial to begin monitoring the casualty's vital signs. This applies whether they're conscious or unconscious. Maintaining communication with the casualty, even if they're unconscious, by calmly explaining your actions is paramount.

Should you notice any significant alterations in the casualty's vital signs during monitoring, don't hesitate to contact emergency services again at 911.

Where should you assess vital signs?

Vital signs are most accurately assessed in the core area of the individual. This core area typically spans from the head down to the thighs. Within this central region lie critical components of our physiology—the brain, heart, lungs, vital organs, and major blood vessels. In times of injury or illness, changes in stability often manifest in the core as the body prioritizes protection of these vital organs and the brain. This physiological response can sometimes lead to a condition known as shock, where the body restricts peripheral circulation to safeguard the core.

How to Document Vital Signs for an Injured Person

Consistently monitor vital signs, noting them down at regular intervals—every 15 minutes or even more frequently, especially for children and the elderly, who may experience rapid changes in condition. When documenting your observations, refrain from using subjective terms like "normal" or "same as me," as everyone's baseline differs. Instead, opt for descriptive terms such as "skin feels warm and dry," "breathing is regular," or "pulse is strong." By employing precise language, you provide clearer and more informative records, aiding in accurate assessment and ongoing care for the casualty.

Spotting Signs: Understanding Vital Signs in Your Patient

Color Check: In the world of first aid, paying attention to the color of your patient's skin can offer valuable insights into their condition. A healthy individual typically sports a rosy pink hue, visible inside the lips, gums, or eyelids—a sign of well-oxygenated blood coursing through their veins.

However, deviations from this norm could indicate trouble. A bluish or grayish tinge may signal low oxygen levels, while a bright cherry red might hint at carbon monoxide poisoning. On the other hand, a yellowish tone could point to jaundice. Remember, as a first aider, your role isn't to diagnose but to observe and document what you see in the moment.

Check the Refill: Another useful technique is the capillary refill test, which assesses peripheral circulation. Press firmly on the patient's cheekbone or forehead, then release and watch how quickly the area refills with blood. Ideally, it should take 1-2 seconds. This test offers valuable insights into circulation changes, particularly in the elderly and young patients. It's also handy for comparing the refill rate of an injured limb with that of an uninjured one—a slower refill in the injured limb could indicate compromised blood flow and warrants further attention.

Temperature Monitoring in First Aid

Our body's normal temperature hovers around 37°C, a vital sign often overlooked in basic first aid kits. But fear not, as you possess a built-in thermometer—your hand! Here's a simple technique: place your hand at the top of your spine, behind your collar, until it reaches the same temperature as your core. Voila! You've got your very own calibrated thermometer.

Now, use this 'calibrated' hand to check your casualty's temperature in the same spot, near the top of their spine. It should feel warm and dry. By regularly comparing your temperature with your casualty's, you can spot any deviations.

Abnormal temperatures can signal underlying issues. Hot and wet may indicate infection, while hot and dry could signal heat stroke. Conversely, cold and wet may point to shock, and cold and dry might suggest hypothermia.

Keep a keen eye on your casualty's temperature, as changes could indicate shock setting in—they might become anxious, cold, and clammy rapidly. Regular monitoring and record-keeping are key to effective first aid response. Stay vigilant, stay prepared!

Breathing

Assessing someone's breathing goes beyond simply checking if they are breathing. It's about understanding the quality, rate, and description of their breaths. Take a moment to observe their breathing closely: listen to the sound, feel the rise and fall of their chest or belly, and note how many breaths they take in 10 seconds. For adults, the average rate is between 12 to 18 breaths per minute.

When documenting their breathing, use descriptive language that accurately reflects what you observe. Normal breathing is typically quiet and regular. However, abnormal breathing may manifest as irregular, gasping, wheezing, raspy, or gurgling. These descriptors are crucial as they help emergency responders assess the situation accurately and provide appropriate guidance over the phone.

Consistently monitor and record the person's breathing pattern to track any changes or improvements over time. By paying attention to these details, you can effectively communicate the condition of the casualty and ensure they receive the necessary assistance in a timely manner.

Pulse

The pulse signifies the heart's beat, measuring both its rate and strength. Where is it located? It's typically found where blood flows through an artery and crosses over a compressed area near the body's surface. Common spots include the neck (carotid pulse) and wrist (radial pulse). Stick to the 'core' area if outdoors or if the person has an injured arm, favoring the neck.

Pulse rate: An average adult's pulse rate ranges from 60-100 beats per minute or 15-25 per 15 seconds. This varies based on fitness and size.

Pulse strength: Alongside rate, note the pulse's strength—strong, weak, rapid, or bounding. Avoid pressing too hard and be attentive to both strength and rate. Some may have an irregular pulse rate, requiring a full-minute count. Describing pulse strength aids emergency services.

Pulses also exist in other body points, useful for monitoring injuries or compromised blood flow. They include the groin (femoral artery), behind the knee (popliteal artery), ankle joint (posterior tibial artery), and foot (dorsalis pedis artery). Practice finding these points on yourself or others for future reference.

In some cases, checking multiple pulse points is beneficial. Starting from extremities and moving inward provides a comprehensive baseline. Comparing pulses between limbs, like in a broken leg scenario, is also useful.

Struggling to find a pulse? Persist and practice on yourself, friends, and family to build confidence. Once found, mark the pulse for easy relocation and inform emergency services of its location. Regularly monitor and record pulse results. Utilizing a pulse-oximeter to assess pulse and oxygen levels in a casualty can be beneficial in certain situations.

These fingertip devices offer a reasonably accurate reading of both pulse and blood oxygen levels. While they may not match the precision of NHS devices, as long as they are consistent with themselves, they serve as valuable monitoring tools.

However, it's important to note potential limitations. Cold hands or fingers may yield less accurate pulse readings compared to the neck pulse. Additionally, the device's battery level can impact the accuracy of readings. Factors such as nail varnish or stained fingers from smoking can interfere with the device's functionality. In such cases, using a toe for the device may be necessary. Nevertheless, it's crucial for first aiders to maintain the ability to manually assess pulse, rather than relying solely on devices.

Assessing Alertness: The AVPU Method

The AVPU method is a vital tool for first aiders, globally recognized for gauging a casualty's level of alertness. AVPU stands for Alertness, Voice, Pressure, and Unresponsive, providing a simple scale to assess consciousness from fully alert to unresponsive.

A – Alert: If the casualty is alert, they can respond sensibly to questions, maintain eye contact, and follow instructions.

V – Voice: If the casualty only responds to a voice or verbal command, ask them to perform simple actions like opening their eyes, blinking, or smiling.

P – Pressure: Apply gentle pressure while observing the casualty's reaction. They may respond with a groan. Place your thumbs above their collarbone and ask them to open their eyes if they feel the pressure.

U – Unresponsive: If the casualty remains unresponsive to any stimulus, immediately call for help.

Handing Over to Emergency Services: When emergency services arrive, provide them with your record sheet. Consider taking a photo or scanning it for your records before handing it over.

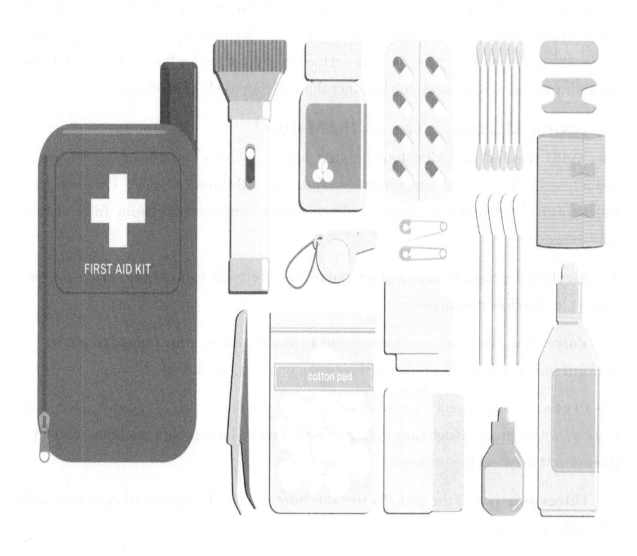

FIRST AID KIT

cotton pad

CHAPTER 2: FIRST AID ESSENTIALS

It's crucial to have a well-equipped first-aid kit readily available in your home. Being prepared with the right supplies can make all the difference in managing emergencies promptly. Ensure you have a first-aid kit both at home and in your vehicle, and remember to pack one when traveling with your family.

You can easily acquire a first aid kit from drugstores or your local Red Cross office, or you can assemble one yourself. When creating your own kit, opt for spacious, durable containers that are easy to carry and open. Consider using plastic tackle boxes or containers typically used for storing art supplies; they're lightweight, feature convenient handles, and provide ample space with separate sections for organization. This way, you'll have everything you need neatly organized and accessible whenever and wherever emergencies strike.

Essential First Aid Supplies

When assembling your first-aid kit, make sure to include these essential items:

- **An Up-to-Date First-Aid Manual**: It's your go-to guide for handling various emergencies effectively.

- **Emergency Phone Numbers List**: Keep a list of important numbers for quick reference during crises.

- **Sterile Gauze Pads**: In various sizes for dressing wounds.

- **Adhesive Tape and Bandages**: Assorted sizes of adhesive bandages (like Band-Aids) and tape for securing dressings.

- **Elastic Bandage and Splint**: Useful for stabilizing fractures or sprains until medical help arrives.

- **Antiseptic Wipes, Soap, and Hand Sanitizer**: For cleaning and disinfecting wounds and hands.

- **Antiseptic Solution**: Such as hydrogen peroxide, for deeper wound cleansing.

- **Sterile Water or Saline Solution**: Along with a large syringe for wound irrigation.

- **Tweezers, Scissors, and Safety Pins**: For handling various tasks, from removing splinters to securing bandages.

- **Disposable Cold Packs and Alcohol Wipes**: For treating injuries and sterilizing equipment.

- **Thermometer and Tooth Preservation Kit**: Essential for monitoring temperatures and preserving knocked-out teeth.

- **Non-Latex Gloves**: At least two pairs for protecting yourself during treatment.

- **Flashlight with Extra Batteries**: To provide illumination in dimly lit areas.

- **Mouthpiece for CPR**: Obtainable from your local Red Cross, crucial for administering CPR.

- **Eye Shield and Eye Wash Solution**: For protecting and cleansing the eyes in case of injury.

Remember to stock up your kit with medications your family might require, including:

- Antibiotic ointment

- Hydrocortisone cream (1%)

- Calamine lotion

- Acetaminophen and ibuprofen

- An antihistamine (anti-itch medicine) such as Benadryl, Zyrtec, Claritin, or store brands

- Extra prescription medications, especially if you're traveling

- Medicine syringes and cups

Once you've got your first-aid kits sorted:

- Take some time to go through the first-aid manual, ensuring you're familiar with how to use the contents effectively.

- It's a good idea to involve your kids if they're old enough, reviewing the key points together. Remember to periodically revisit the manual and ensure it's up to date.

- Keep your first-aid kits stored in a place that's inaccessible to children but easily accessible for adults. Regularly inspect the kits, replacing any missing items or anything that's expired.

- Ensure that babysitters and other caregivers are aware of where the kit is located and how to utilize its contents.

- Don't forget to check the flashlight batteries to ensure they're in working order.

- If you're traveling by air, pack the first-aid kit in your checked luggage. Keep in mind that some items may not be permitted in carry-on bags.

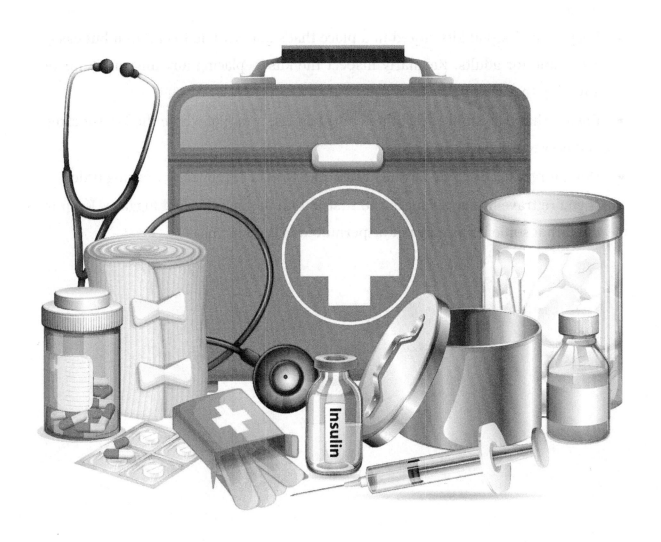

CHAPTER 3: LIFESAVING TECHNIQUES

Mastering first aid lifesaving techniques is paramount for anyone, as it can be the decisive factor between life and death in critical situations. Understanding the core principles of prioritizing safety, assessing victims, and activating emergency services forms the foundation of effective first aid response. By equipping oneself with these lifesaving skills and knowledge, individuals can confidently respond to emergencies, alleviate suffering, and potentially save lives within their communities.

Assessing an unconscious Victim

Unconsciousness describes a state where someone cannot react to stimuli and seems asleep. It could last for just a few seconds, like in fainting, or extend to longer durations. When unconscious, individuals won't react to loud noises or being shaken, and their breathing might cease or pulse weaken. This demands immediate emergency assistance. The quicker they receive first aid, the more favorable their chances become.

How can you tell if someone might lose consciousness soon? Look out for these signs:

- They suddenly can't respond.

- Their speech becomes slurred.

- Their heart starts racing.

- They seem confused.

- They feel dizzy or lightheaded.

When it comes to administering first aid, your initial actions can be critical. If you encounter someone unconscious, your first priority is to assess their breathing.

If they're not breathing, it's imperative to act swiftly. Have someone call 911 or your local emergency services while you prepare to initiate CPR. Every second counts in such situations. On the other hand, if the person is breathing, your focus shifts to ensuring their safety. Gently maneuver them into the recovery position. This simple action not only helps maintain an open airway but also reduces the risk of choking, offering them the best chance of recovery. Remember, in emergencies, quick and decisive action can make all the difference.

When assisting someone who is unconscious but breathing, follow these steps:

1. Position yourself next to them on the floor, kneeling down.

2. Take the arm nearest to you and gently place it so that it forms a right angle with their body, palm facing upward.

3. Place their other hand against the cheek closest to you, keeping it in position.

4. Using your free hand, bend the knee farthest from you, ensuring the foot remains flat on the floor.

5. Help them roll onto their side by gently pulling on the bent knee.

6. Ensure their top arm continues to support their head after rolling them over.

7. Gently tilt their head back and lift their chin to open their airway.

8. Check for any obstructions in their airway.

9. Stay with them, monitoring their condition closely, until emergency help arrives.

If heavy bleeding is present, your immediate priority is to locate the source of the injury and apply direct pressure to the bleeding area. Maintain pressure until the bleeding slows, and professional help arrives. For limb injuries with significant bleeding, consider applying a tourniquet above the wound site while awaiting medical assistance. Remember to follow proper tourniquet application techniques for optimal effectiveness.

In cases of severe wounds, take these steps:

1. Elevate the injured body part (except for head injuries) to reduce blood flow.
2. Apply moderate pressure to the wound to control bleeding (except for eye injuries).
3. Assist the individual in lying down to prevent falls and minimize the risk of further injury in case of fainting.

What leads to unconsciousness?

Unconsciousness can arise from significant health issues or injuries, as well as complications stemming from substance abuse, like drug or alcohol misuse.

Typical triggers for unconsciousness encompass various scenarios:

- Involvement in a car accident

- Experiencing severe blood loss

- Suffering a blow to the chest or head

- Overdosing on drugs

- Falling victim to alcohol poisoning

Furthermore, temporary unconsciousness, often referred to as fainting, occurs due to sudden bodily changes. Common triggers for temporary loss of consciousness include:

- Low blood sugar levels

- Dropping blood pressure

- Syncope, which occurs when inadequate blood flow reaches the brain

- Neurologic syncope, induced by seizures, strokes, or transient ischemic attacks (TIAs)

- Dehydration

- Irregular heart rhythms

- Experiencing strain or hyperventilation

CPR and AED

Performing CPR on someone who isn't breathing can be a crucial lifeline until emergency services arrive. Knowing when and how to administer CPR is essential. CPR sustains blood circulation in the absence of professional medical assistance, potentially saving a life. Even without formal first aid training, anyone can make a difference by following CPR protocols.

Immediate CPR significantly increases the likelihood of survival when initiated promptly after cardiac arrest. In fact, it can double or even triple the chances of survival. By understanding CPR's importance and being prepared to act decisively, individuals can play a vital role in the chain of survival.

CPR, Step-by-Step:

Let's break down CPR into two crucial stages: preparation and execution.

Preparation:

1. **Call 911**: Safety first. Scan the surroundings for potential dangers like traffic or debris. Check on the person in need by gently tapping their shoulder and asking, "Are you OK?" If there is no response, promptly call 911 or ask someone nearby to make the call. Also, if available, enlist someone to fetch an AED machine from nearby establishments.

2. **Positioning and Airway**: Gently lay the individual on their back and position yourself next to them. Slightly tilt their head back by lifting their chin, ensuring an open airway. Peek inside their mouth for any obstructions like food or vomit. If you spot something, remove it carefully. However, if it's lodged tightly, avoid pushing it deeper.

3. **Breathing Check**: Now, listen closely. Place your ear near their mouth and nose, listening for breath sounds for no more than 10 seconds. If you don't detect any breathing or hear only sporadic gasps, it's time to initiate CPR. Remember, if the person is unconscious but still breathing, don't perform CPR. Instead, if they don't seem to have a spinal injury, gently place them in the recovery position while keeping a close eye on their breathing. Be prepared to resume CPR if their breathing ceases.

To perform CPR effectively, follow these steps:

Step 4. Chest Compressions:

Place one hand over the other and lock them together. Position your hands at the center of the chest, just below the nipples. Now, with straight arms, press down firmly using the heel of your hand. Aim for a depth of at least 2 inches, and maintain a steady rhythm, delivering around 100 compressions per minute. Allow the chest to fully rise between compressions, ensuring effective circulation.

Step 5. Rescue Breaths:

Ensure the person's airway is clear, then gently tilt their head back and lift their chin to open the air passage. Pinch their nose shut, form a tight seal over their mouth with yours, and deliver two full breaths to inflate their lungs. If you don't see their chest rise after the first breath, readjust their head position before trying again. If their chest still doesn't rise after the second attempt, they may be experiencing an obstruction.

Step 6. Repeat:

Continue the cycle of 30 chest compressions followed by two rescue breaths until the person shows signs of breathing or until help arrives. If an Automated External Defibrillator (AED) becomes available, keep performing CPR until the device is ready for use. Your persistence and prompt actions can make a life-saving difference.

CPR for Children and Infants

Performing CPR on children and infants requires slightly different steps compared to adults. Here's how:

Preparation Steps

Before administering CPR to an infant or child, follow these preparation steps:

Step 1: Assess the Situation and Call for Help

Start by assessing the surroundings for any potential hazards. Then, check the child or infant for signs of responsiveness. For children, gently tap their shoulder and ask, "Are you OK?" For infants, stimulate them by gently flicking the sole of their foot.

If you're alone with the child and they're unresponsive, provide two minutes of care before dialing 911. If there's a bystander present, instruct them to call 911 while you provide care.

If available, assign a bystander to locate an AED machine, commonly found in offices and public buildings.

If the child responds, still call 911 if any life-threatening conditions are evident.

Step 2: Position and Open the Airway

Carefully lay the child or infant on their back and kneel beside their chest. Gently tilt their head backward by lifting their chin.

Open their mouth and check for obstructions like food or vomit. If you can easily remove the obstruction, do so. However, if it's not easily dislodged, refrain from touching it to prevent pushing it deeper into the airway.

Step 3: Check for Breathing

Place your ear near their mouth and listen for approximately 10 seconds. If you don't detect breathing or only hear sporadic gasps, initiate CPR.

Note that infants may exhibit irregular breathing patterns, which is usually normal.

Continue monitoring their breathing, ready to administer CPR if breathing ceases.

Now, let's go through the steps for performing CPR on a child or infant:

Step 4: Giving Rescue Breaths

If the child or infant isn't breathing, it's crucial to administer two rescue breaths while ensuring their head is tilted back and chin raised.

For a child, gently close their nostrils and place your mouth over theirs, giving two breaths.

For an infant, cover their nose and mouth with your mouth and blow for about a second to expand their chest. Then, provide two rescue breaths.

If they remain unresponsive, proceed to chest compressions.

Step 5: Chest Compressions

Position yourself beside the child or infant.

For a child, use one hand. Position your hand's heel on their sternum, located at the chest's center, between and slightly below their nipples. Apply firm and rapid pressure, about 2 inches deep, at a rate of at least 100 compressions per minute.

For an infant, employ two fingers. Place them at the chest's center, between and slightly below the nipples, and perform 30 compressions swiftly, about 1.5 inches deep.

Step 6: Repeat

Continue the sequence of rescue breaths and chest compressions until the child shows signs of breathing or until medical help arrives.

Knowing when to administer CPR can be critical in emergency situations. For adults, initiate CPR when they're not breathing at all. With children or infants, it's necessary when they're not breathing normally. Always resort to CPR if there's no response when attempting to communicate or stimulate them.

CPR is vital as it ensures oxygenated blood reaches the brain, preventing potential brain damage or death within a short timeframe of approximately 8 minutes without oxygen.

Several scenarios may necessitate CPR:

- Cardiac arrest or heart attack

- Choking

- Road traffic accidents

- Near-drowning incidents

- Suffocation

- Poisoning

- Drug or alcohol overdoses

- Smoke inhalation

- Electrocution

- Suspected sudden infant death syndrome

Remember, only administer CPR if the individual isn't breathing (or breathing abnormally in children and infants) and if their blood isn't circulating. Always confirm the lack of response before initiating CPR procedures.

AED

Have you ever wondered about those mysterious AEDs popping up in offices and public spaces, if you have, then you're not alone. With their increasing presence, more folks are naturally curious about what they are and why they're there. So, what exactly is an AED?

Well, an AED stands for **Automated External Defibrillator**. It's essentially a device designed to assist individuals experiencing sudden cardiac arrest. Despite its sophisticated functions, it's surprisingly user-friendly. The AED can analyze the heart's rhythm and, if needed, administer an electrical shock, known as defibrillation, to help the heart restore a normal rhythm.

How does an AED work?

Sudden cardiac arrest occurs when the heart experiences irregular rhythms, depriving the body of oxygen and blood flow to critical organs like the brain. Automated External Defibrillators (AEDs) are designed to swiftly identify these irregularities and administer a controlled electric shock, called defibrillation, to restore the heart's normal rhythm.

The Heart and Stroke Foundation of USA highlights that immediate AED use, coupled with cardiopulmonary resuscitation (CPR), can significantly enhance survival rates by 75% or more. AEDs come in various types and are manufactured by different companies. However, regardless of brand or model, they operate similarly once activated.

Each AED unit comprises adhesive pads with electrodes (sensors) placed on the chest of a person experiencing cardiac arrest. These electrodes analyze the heart's rhythm and relay the data to the AED's processor to determine if a controlled electric shock is necessary. Upon detecting abnormal rhythms, the device delivers an automatic, controlled shock through the electrodes to restore normal heart function.

Types of AEDs

There are two primary types Automated External Defibrillators (AEDs)

i.   Fully automatic AED

ii. Semi-automatic AED

Fully Automatic AED: With this type of AED, once the electrode pads are connected and the device is powered on, it takes charge. It analyzes the person's heart rhythm and, if a shock is deemed necessary, it administers it automatically following a prompt or countdown period, requiring no action from the rescuer. This hands-free functionality makes it particularly appealing for individuals with limited or no training, as it demands minimal user interaction.

Semi-automatic AED: In contrast, the semi-automatic AED relies on the rescuer to initiate the shock by pressing a button. Like its fully automatic counterpart, it assesses the heart rhythm and decides on the need for a shock, but it requires the rescuer to follow its instructions to administer the shock manually. The advantage here lies in the rescuer's ability to exert more control over the device, including the option to delay the shock if circumstances warrant it.

How to Use AED

Using an AED (Automated External Defibrillator) can be crucial when assisting a non-breathing adult or child weighing at least 55 pounds and aged eight years or older. Before anything else, ensure the surroundings are safe for both you and the individual in distress. If there are any potential risks, like water nearby, move them to a safer spot. Also, take a moment to remove any adhesive patches, such as those for nicotine, birth control, nitroglycerin, or pain relief, from the person's body.

Next, power up the AED by pressing the on/off button. To properly attach the electrode pads, expose the person's chest by removing any clothing or jewelry covering it, and if the chest is wet, gently wipe it dry. Be cautious not to place the pads directly over a pacemaker. Following the visual or vocal instructions on the AED, place one pad on the upper right side of the chest, just below the collarbone, and the other on the lower left side, below the left armpit.

Once the pads are in place, allow the AED to analyze the heart rhythm. Make sure no one is touching the person, and loudly announce "CLEAR!" before delivering a shock if advised. Remember, if the AED is fully automatic, it will administer the shock automatically after prompting you.

Immediately after a shock, initiate CPR with 30 chest compressions and two rescue breaths. The AED will guide you through this process until emergency medical services arrive. Following these steps ensures you're playing a vital role in potentially saving someone's life during a critical situation.

Assisting a Choking Victim

Choking occurs when an object obstructs the throat or windpipe, impeding the flow of air. Among adults, food is often the culprit, while small objects pose risks for young children. It's a critical, life-threatening situation that deprives the brain of oxygen. Acting swiftly with first aid is crucial if you or someone else is choking.

Look out for these signs indicating choking:

- Clutching one or both hands to the throat

- Exhibiting panic, shock, or confusion in their expression

- Inability to vocalize

- Breathing that sounds strained or noisy

- Emitting squeaky sounds while attempting to breathe

- Coughing, which may be weak or forceful

- Skin, lips, and nails taking on a bluish or grayish hue

- Loss of consciousness

If someone is choking and can cough forcefully, it's best to let them continue coughing. Often, coughing can naturally dislodge the obstructing object, providing relief without needing further intervention. It's important to stay calm and supportive in such situations, reassuring the person and encouraging them to keep coughing until the object is expelled. If someone finds themselves unable to cough, speak, or exhibit forceful expressions like crying or laughing, immediate first aid is crucial.

Following the recommendations of the American Red Cross:

- Start with five back blows. Position yourself just behind and to the side of an adult who's choking. For a child, kneel down behind them. Provide support by placing your arm across their chest and bending them over at the waist, facing the ground. Administer five firm strikes between their shoulder blades using the heel of your hand.
- Proceed with five abdominal thrusts if back blows fail to dislodge the obstruction, commonly known as the **Heimlich Maneuver**.
- Repeat the sequence of five back blows and five abdominal thrusts until the blockage is cleared.
- While some resources solely emphasize the abdominal thrust technique, it's permissible to omit back blows if you haven't been trained in this method. Both approaches are deemed suitable for adults and children over the age of one.

When you need to perform abdominal thrusts on someone else:

- Stand behind them. If it's a child, kneel down behind them for better reach. Position one foot slightly in front of the other to maintain balance.
- Wrap your arms around their waist and gently tip them forward.
- With one hand, form a fist and place it just above their navel.
- Hold your fist with your other hand and deliver a quick, upward thrust into their stomach (abdomen), aiming to dislodge the obstruction. For children, be sure to use gentle yet firm pressure to avoid causing harm.
- Administer five abdominal thrusts, then check to see if the blockage has cleared. Repeat the process if necessary.
- If you're the sole rescuer, begin with back blows and abdominal thrusts before dialing 911 or your local emergency number for assistance. If someone else is present, have them make the emergency call while you administer first aid.
- Should the person lose consciousness, transition to standard CPR with chest compressions and rescue breaths.

If the individual is pregnant or if you find it challenging to encircle the abdomen with your arms, opt for chest thrusts:

- Position your hands at the bottom of the breastbone, right above where the lowest ribs meet.
- Apply firm pressure to the chest with a swift thrust, mimicking the action of the Heimlich maneuver.
- Continue with this motion until the obstruction is dislodged from the airway.

If you find yourself needing to clear the airway of an unconscious person

- the first step is to carefully lower them to the floor, ensuring their back is flat and their arms are at their sides.
- Next, take a moment to assess the airway. If you can see the object causing the blockage, gently remove it using your finger. However, if you can't see the object, avoid blindly reaching in, as you might accidentally push it deeper, especially with children.
- If the person still isn't responding after clearing the airway, it's time to initiate CPR. If the airway remains blocked, incorporate chest compressions, similar to those used in CPR, to dislodge the obstruction. Remember, administer only two rescue breaths per cycle, and be sure to regularly check the mouth for any remaining obstructions.

Alright, let's talk about helping a choking infant under the age of 1.

- First, find a comfortable spot to sit, then place the infant face down on your forearm, making sure your forearm is resting on your thigh. Hold the infant's chin and jaw to support their head, making sure it's lower than their trunk.
- Now, gently but firmly thump the infant's back five times in the middle, using the heel of your hand. Remember to point your fingers upwards to avoid hitting the back of their head. These thumps, along with gravity, should hopefully dislodge the blockage.
- If the infant still isn't breathing, carefully turn them face up on your forearm, ensuring their head is lower than their trunk. With your fingers just below the nipple

line, give five gentle but firm chest compressions, pressing down about 1 1/2 inches. Make sure to let the chest rise between each compression.

- Repeat the back thumps and chest compressions if necessary, and don't hesitate to call for emergency medical help. If the airway clears but the infant still isn't breathing, it's time to start infant CPR.

If you find yourself alone and in the frightening situation of choking, it's crucial to act swiftly. First things first: dial 911 or your local emergency number immediately. Then, focus on freeing the obstruction with abdominal thrusts, commonly known as the Heimlich maneuver.

Here's how you do it:

- Position your fist just above your navel.
- Firmly grip your fist with your other hand.
- Bend forward, utilizing a sturdy surface like a countertop or chair for support.
- With a quick, forceful motion, push your fist inward and upward, aiming to dislodge the obstructing object.
- By following these steps, you're taking decisive action to clear your airway and potentially save your own life.

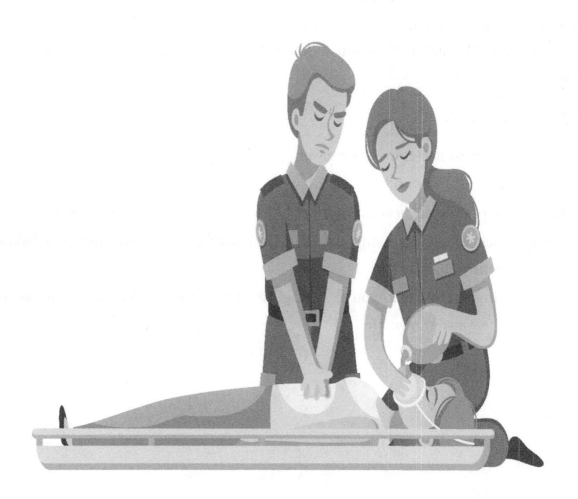

CHAPTER 4: TREATING MINOR INJURIES

W e would be taking a look at the essential techniques for addressing common minor injuries effectively. Whether it's a small cut, a mild burn, or a sprained ankle, knowing how to provide prompt and appropriate care can aid in a quick recovery and prevent complications.

This section covers a range of topics, including wound cleaning and dressing, managing burns and scalds, handling sprains and strains, and treating minor allergic reactions. The section is designed to equip you with practical skills and tips to confidently manage these injuries at home or in emergency situations.

Managing Cuts, Grazes, and Wounds

Cuts

Cuts and wounds result from a break in body tissue, caused by external actions like bruising, cuts, or hematomas. They are very common, with most people experiencing them at some point in their lives. While some wounds are minor and can be treated at home, others are more severe and require immediate medical attention to prevent complications.

What are Wounds?

Wounds refer to injuries that damage the body and can occur due to falls, accidents, or contact with objects. Wounds are injuries that break the skin or other body tissues, such as scrapes, punctures, cuts, and scratches. Minor wounds can often be treated at home, but more severe or infected wounds may require initial first aid followed by medical attention from a doctor. It's crucial to seek medical care for deep wounds to prevent excessive bleeding or hemorrhaging. Thoroughly cleaning wounds is essential to prevent infection and promote healing.

Types of Cuts and Wounds

Abrasions

An abrasion, commonly known as a scrape, occurs when the skin is rubbed off due to friction. This creates a break in the skin, often resulting in slight bleeding and discomfort. Abrasions typically occur accidentally when something impacts or drags against the skin.

Imagine an abrasion like using sandpaper to remove paint from an object. The rough texture of the sandpaper rubbing against the object strips away layers of paint, much like how an abrasion removes layers of skin. This injury affects only the outermost layers of the skin, similar to the surface layers of paint being removed from an object.

Types of Abrasions

There are three types of Abrasions

1. Linear Abrasion (Scratch): A linear abrasion is like a scratch on the skin, caused by a sharp, pointed object such as a thorn.

2. Grazed Abrasion (Brushed Abrasion): This type of abrasion results from the skin coming into contact with or sliding across a rough surface, covering a larger area like a skinned knee.

3. Patterned Abrasion: This occurs when an object forcefully contacts the skin and leaves a mark that matches its shape and size. For instance, cat scratches leave nail-shaped wounds reflecting the claws' size and shape.

How to Treat an Abrasion

Treating an abrasion involves proper wound care, which you can do at home following these steps:

- Clean the Wound: Gently wash the abrasion with soap and water to remove dirt and bacteria.
- Remove Debris: Use tweezers to carefully remove visible debris, like small stones or dirt. Be careful not to force out embedded debris. If the wound has a lot of debris or is deep, seek medical help to avoid further injury.
- Dry the Wound: Pat the area dry with a clean washcloth after washing.
- Apply Antibiotic Ointment: Use a topical antibiotic ointment to prevent infection.
- Cover the Wound: Use a bandage or wound dressing to protect the abrasion. For smaller abrasions, a bandage may not be necessary.

- Daily Care: Clean and re-dress the wound daily until it heals. Always use a fresh bandage each time.

- If the abrasion is large, or if you experience severe symptoms, seek immediate medical attention. Stitches may be required for larger wounds.

- For animal-related abrasions, your healthcare provider may recommend a tetanus shot or antibiotics as preventive measures against infection. Seek medical attention within 24 hours of an animal bite or scratch to minimize infection risk.

- Avoid picking at the abrasion to promote faster healing and reduce the risk of infection. Resist the urge to peel off scabs or scratch the wound, as this can worsen the injury and introduce bacteria.

Laceration

A laceration is an injury that occurs when tissue is torn, often resulting from accidents involving tools, machinery, or knives. This type of wound is characterized by deep cuts that can lead to significant bleeding. The forceful tearing of tissue can cause damage not only to the skin but also to underlying structures such as muscles, tendons, bones, and blood vessels in the vicinity.

A laceration occurs when the skin, tissue, or muscle is torn or cut open due to impact from an object. Lacerations can vary in depth, length, and width. Repairing a laceration involves cleaning, preparing, and closing the wound. Minor lacerations, which are shallow, small, clean, and not bleeding heavily, may not require medical attention and can be managed with antibiotic ointment and a bandage. However, most lacerations need to be repaired.

Proper cleaning and preparation of a laceration are essential to prevent infection and minimize scarring. Cleaning removes dirt and germs that can cause infection. Regardless of the closure technique used, cleaning is performed in the same way. Preparation involves smoothing out jagged edges to promote less noticeable scarring and is done as needed.

Types of Laceration

1. **Contused Laceration**: This type of laceration occurs beneath the skin's surface, causing trauma to the soft tissues without breaking the skin. It typically results from blunt impacts to bony areas, compressing the tissues against the bone and leaving the skin intact. When the edges of the laceration are abraded, it's also known as an abraded laceration.

2. **Split Laceration**: Also called a slit laceration, this occurs when the skin is crushed between two hard objects, such as bones or a hard surface. The skin splits open due to the pressure.

3. **Incised Laceration**: Characterized by clean, sharp wound edges without tissue bridging or excessive skin damage. It can be mistaken for other types, so close examination is necessary. Common sites include the scalp, eyebrows, and forehead.

4. **Stretch Laceration**: Caused by overstretching of the skin, leading the skin layer to protrude like a flap when fixed in position. These lacerations can occur, for example, when someone is struck by a moving vehicle.

5. **Tear Laceration**: Occurs when the skin rubs against irregular or semi-sharp objects, tearing deeper at the beginning and shallower towards the end of the wound. For instance, contact with a car door handle can cause this type of injury.

6. **Cut Lacerations**: Result from heavy, sharp-edged instruments crushing and splitting a broad area of the skin. These injuries involve trauma from both cutting and tearing of tissues, leading to bleeding.

Treatment of Lacerated Wound

Lacerations, regardless of their severity, require prompt attention and repair due to several important reasons:

- Even after cleaning, dirt and debris may persist within the wound.
- When a laceration penetrates deeper than 1/4th or 1/8th into the skin, it requires repair.
- If muscle, fat, tendon, or bone is visible beyond the skin, prompt repair is necessary.

- If bleeding continues for more than twenty minutes post-injury, it's crucial to address and repair the wound.
- Wounds near sensitive regions like the eyes or areas subject to increased stress require immediate attention.
- Deeper injuries are more likely to scar; repair helps minimize scarring.

Steps for Treatment:

- Stop bleeding by applying direct pressure to the wound.
- Clean the wound with warm water or a saline solution to remove debris and minimize infection risk.
- Deep or joint lacerations should be closed within 12 hours of injury to reduce infection risk. Options for closure include bandages, cyanoacrylate glue, staples, or sutures (preferably absorbable to reduce scarring and infection risk).
- Monitor healing progress; seek professional care if the wound doesn't heal properly, especially for deeper or severe injuries. Minor injuries typically heal well with proper cleaning and closure.

Incision

An incision refers to a clean, sharp cut in the skin caused by a sharp object. For example, accidentally cutting oneself with a kitchen knife or scissors can result in this type of injury. Another type of incision is made intentionally during a surgical procedure, where a doctor cuts through the skin to access internal body parts for medical treatment.

Cuts, like those from a knife while preparing food, can be painful and may result in infection if not managed correctly. It's important to understand which cuts can be handled at home and which require medical attention.

Incision wounds vary in severity, categorized as superficial or deep. Superficial cuts only penetrate the outer layer of skin, while deep cuts extend beyond 1 cm and can impact tendons, muscles, ligaments, nerves, blood vessels, and even bones. Knowing the depth of the cut helps determine the appropriate course of action for treatment and healing.

First Aid for Incisions

You can manage superficial wounds at home with proper care and attention. Follow these steps for effective wound treatment:

1. Wash your hands thoroughly with soap and water before handling the wound.

2. Use clean running water to gently rinse the wound. Avoid using harsh antiseptics like hydrogen peroxide or alcohol, especially for larger or deeper cuts, as they can cause skin irritation.

3. Use a clean cloth or sterile gauze to cover the wound. For larger wounds, apply sterile gauze and secure with a bandage. Minor wounds can be left uncovered to heal naturally.

4. Apply aloe vera gel to superficial wounds to aid in healing. Use commercial aloe vera gel or extract gel directly from a fresh aloe plant.

5. Take over-the-counter pain relievers such as paracetamol for pain relief. Steer clear of aspirin, as it may increase the likelihood of bleeding.

6. If the wound is bruised or swollen, apply a cold compress (ice wrapped in a cloth) to the affected area. Avoid placing ice directly on the wound.

7. Maintain the wound's cleanliness and dryness for 5-7 days. Avoid picking at scabs or itching the wound.

8. During the healing period, avoid smoking, alcohol, and excessive stress, as they can impede the healing process.

For deep wounds, such as those caused by cutting, immediate medical attention is crucial. These wounds can be identified by visible layers beneath the skin and significant bleeding, especially if large blood vessels are affected. Seek medical help promptly at the nearest healthcare facility—do not wait longer than 6 hours regardless of the wound's size or depth. Delaying treatment can lead to shock due to continued bleeding or severe infection.

Additionally, certain wound conditions require a doctor's attention:

1. Extremely dirty wounds that are difficult to clean.

2. Wounds from scratches or animal bites, especially on sensitive areas like the face or near joints.

3. Injuries from accidents or impacts with subtle signs of internal bleeding.

4. Signs of infection such as fever, redness, swelling, pus, or persistent pain.

5. Wounds in patients with diabetes, blood clotting disorders, on blood-thinning medications, or undergoing chemotherapy.

6. Excessive or uncontrollable bleeding lasting more than 10 minutes after applying pressure.

7. Persistent pain, numbness, or delayed healing of wounds.

During recovery, prioritize self-care by eating well, getting enough rest, staying hydrated, avoiding smoking, and limiting alcohol consumption to support healing. If you have concerns about a wound, do not hesitate to consult a healthcare professional.

Puncture

A puncture is a small hole made by a sharp, pointed object like a nail. In certain cases, even a bullet can cause a puncture wound. Although puncture wounds may not bleed much, they can pose serious risks because they have the potential to harm internal organs.

Treating a Puncture Wound

1. Begin by washing your hands thoroughly to prevent infection.

2. Apply gentle pressure using a clean bandage or cloth to stop any bleeding.

3. Rinse the wound with clear water for 5 to 10 minutes. If dirt or debris remains, use a washcloth to gently scrub it off. Seek medical attention if you can't remove all the dirt or debris.

4. Use a thin layer of antibiotic cream or ointment (such as Neosporin or Polysporin) on the wound. Reapply the antibiotic during dressing changes for the first two days. If you develop a rash, discontinue use and consult a healthcare provider. For those allergic to antibiotic ointments, petroleum jelly (Vaseline) can be used.

5. Keep the wound covered with a bandage to protect it and keep it clean.

6. Replace the bandage daily or whenever it becomes wet or dirty.

7. Watch for signs of infection, such as increasing pain, pus, swelling, or fever. Redness can be difficult to detect on darker skin tones; seek medical attention if you notice any unusual changes or signs of infection.

When to Seek Emergency Help:

It's important to seek immediate medical attention if your wound:

- Continues to bleed despite applying firm pressure for an extended period.

- Results from an animal or human bite.

- Is deep and contaminated with dirt.

- Is caused by a metal object.

- Is deep and located on the head, neck, scrotum, chest, or abdomen.

- Occurs over a joint and could be deep.

- Is the result of an assault or attempted suicide.

When to Contact Your Doctor:

Contact your doctor if your wound exhibits signs of infection, such as:

- Fever.

- Inflammation, enlargement, elevated temperature, or escalating discomfort surrounding the injury.

- Foul odor emanating from the wound.

- Pus draining from the wound.

- Red streaks around the wound or extending up your arm or leg.

If you haven't received a tetanus shot within the past five years and the wound is deep or contaminated, your healthcare provider may recommend a booster. It's important to receive the booster shot within 48 hours of the injury.

If the wound was caused by a cat or dog, confirm that the animal's rabies vaccination is up to date. For wounds caused by wild animals, consult your doctor to determine which animals are most likely to carry rabies.

Avulsion

An avulsion occurs when the skin is partially or completely torn away due to severe accidents, such as car crashes, gunshot wounds, or exposure to explosions. Avulsions often result in heavy bleeding, which can lead to serious complications that threaten life.

There are various types of avulsion wounds:

1. Avulsion Fracture: This occurs when a piece of bone attached to a ligament or tendon is forcefully pulled away from the rest of the bone.

2. Brachial Plexus Avulsion: In this injury, the root of nerves in the brachial plexus, located along the spinal cord and neck, becomes detached from the spinal cord.

3. Ear Avulsion: Ear avulsions involve the separation of some or all of the outer part of the ear from the head.

4. Eyelid Avulsion: This occurs when some or all of the eyelid tissue is torn away, affecting either the upper or lower eyelid.

5. Nail Avulsion: Nail avulsions happen when part or all of the nail is torn or removed from the nail bed. Surgical procedures may sometimes be required, especially for chronic ingrown toenails.

6. Surgical Avulsion: This involves the permanent removal of a body part through a surgical procedure.

7. Tooth Avulsion: Tooth avulsion refers to the complete removal of a tooth from its socket, typically with the root intact. Note that this does not include the natural loss of baby teeth.

Here are the steps for providing first aid for an avulsion injury:

- If you're not the injured person, prioritize your safety by practicing universal precautions and wearing personal protective equipment if available. Stay clear of the cause of the injury and only intervene if it's safe to do so. Remember, you can't help if you become injured yourself.

- Apply direct pressure and elevate the injured area to control bleeding. Use a clean, absorbent dressing or any available clean cloth to apply pressure to the open wound. Direct pressure helps the wound clot and stops the bleeding. Even if the wound exposes muscle or fat tissue, continue applying direct pressure. Avoid using a tourniquet unless bleeding cannot be controlled and medical help will be delayed.

- Cleanse the wound using water or saline solution. Ideally, use sterile irrigation for cleaning. Keep in mind that cleaning the wound may cause some bleeding, which is acceptable as long as it remains minimal. If bleeding was difficult to stop initially and you're concerned about it becoming unmanageable during cleaning, you can skip this step and wait for professional help.

- If the tissue (skin, fat, muscle) is partially torn, attempt to replace the flap and cover the wound. For completely separated tissue, collect it if available and bring it to the emergency department or give it to first responders upon their arrival.

How to Generally Treat Cuts and Wounds

Minor wounds are typically manageable at home, but deeper or more serious injuries may necessitate professional medical attention. Follow these steps for first aid treatment of cuts and wounds:

1. Prior to tending to an open wound, always wash your hands thoroughly to minimize the risk of infection and maintain wound cleanliness.

2. If the wound is deep and bleeding profusely (e.g., lacerations or avulsions), staunch the bleeding immediately by applying gentle pressure with a clean cloth or bandage. Elevate the wound to help control bleeding until it ceases.

3. Once bleeding is under control, rinse the wound with clean water for at least five minutes to remove dirt and debris. Washing with soap and water is advisable to further clean the wound.

4. Use a topical antiseptic to disinfect the wound and reduce the risk of infection.

5. Cover the wound with a sterile gauze pad and dressing, securing it with adhesive tape. Minor scrapes or abrasions may not require covering.

6. For deep wounds with heavy bleeding, promptly refer the individual to a physician or hospital. Such injuries may necessitate suturing or other surgical interventions.

7. Be vigilant for signs of hypovolemic shock in individuals with significant bleeding. Look for paleness, bluish skin coloration, rapid and weak pulse, irregular breathing, and overall weakness.

Grazes

A graze wound is a type of injury to the skin where the topmost layer of the skin (epidermis) is scraped off or abraded due to friction against a rough surface. This type of injury is typically shallow and does not penetrate deeply into the skin or underlying tissues.

Graze wounds often result from falls or accidents where the skin rubs against a hard or rough surface, such as pavement or gravel. They can appear as raw, red areas with minor bleeding and are commonly painful due to exposed nerve endings in the damaged skin.

Graze wounds are generally considered minor injuries that can usually be managed with simple first aid measures, such as cleaning the wound with mild soap and water, applying an antiseptic ointment to prevent infection, and covering the area with a sterile bandage to protect it while it heals. If the wound shows signs of infection or does not heal properly, medical attention may be needed.

First Aid for Graze

You can manage a cut or graze on your own by following a few simple steps. Start by stopping any bleeding, cleaning the wound thoroughly, and then covering it with a plaster or dressing. This helps to prevent infection.

If the wound is painful, you can take over-the-counter painkillers like paracetamol or ibuprofen (avoid giving aspirin to children under 16). These steps will aid in healing and reduce discomfort associated with minor injuries.

Managing Heavy Bleeding

- Check the wound and ensure there's no debris lodged in it.

- If the wound is clear, apply firm pressure using a bandage or clean cloth (like a tea towel) for 10 minutes.

- If an object is stuck in the wound, avoid removing it. Instead, apply pressure on either side of the object to close the wound edges together.

- For wounds on the hand or arm, elevate the affected limb above heart level. For lower limb wounds, lie down and elevate the limb.

- Once bleeding stops, securely wrap a new bandage over the initial one.

- If bleeding persists, maintain pressure by adding another bandage and continue applying firm pressure for another 10 minutes.

How to Dress and Clean a Graze

1. Wash and dry your hands thoroughly. Use disposable gloves if available.

2. Rinse the wound with bottled or tap water, or use sterile wipes to gently clean the area. Avoid cleaning the wound with antiseptic.

3. Use soap and water or antiseptic to clean the skin around the wound, ensuring it's free from dirt or germs.

4. Pat the area dry using a clean gauze swab or a clean tea towel to avoid leaving moisture that can promote infection.

5. Use a sterile dressing or plaster to cover the wound, providing protection and allowing it to heal.

6. Keep the dressing clean by changing it regularly based on the wound's condition. Once the wound has closed after a few days, you can remove the dressing.

When to seek for Medical Help

1. If a wound contains soil, pus, or body fluids, or remains dirty after cleaning.

2. If you were bitten by a person or a wild or stray animal.

3. If a cut appears swollen, red, and increasingly painful, or if pus is present.

4. If a cut is larger than approximately 5 cm (2 inches) in length.

5. If you've sustained a cut and also feel generally unwell or have a high temperature.

In case of any of these situations, calling 911 is advisable.

Handling Sprains and Strains

Sprain

Joints are held stable by a joint capsule and reinforced by strong bands of connective tissue known as ligaments. These supportive structures, often referred to as passive or non-contractile supports, play a key role in maintaining joint stability. Surrounding the entire joint is a membrane containing synovial fluid, which acts as a lubricant to nourish the joint and absorb impact, providing additional cushioning. A sprain occurs when there is damage involving tearing of the ligaments, the joint capsule, or both.

Common areas susceptible to sprains include the thumb, ankle, and knee. These injuries can result from sudden twisting or stretching of the joint beyond its normal range of motion, leading to pain, swelling, and reduced joint function.

Strains

Muscles extend over joints and attach to bones through tendons. They can span either a single joint (single-joint muscles) or multiple joints (multi-joint muscles). When muscles contract, they shorten and exert force on their tendon attachment points on bones, thereby causing joint movement. Multi-joint muscles, such as the hamstrings, quadriceps, and the large calf muscle known as the gastrocnemius, are more prone to injury compared to single-joint muscles. Damage to these muscles or their tendons is referred to as a strain. Common areas where strains occur include the calf, groin, and hamstring.

First Aid for Sprain and Strain

1. Reduce Swelling with RICE Therapy RICE stands for:

   - **Rest**: Take it easy and avoid putting any weight on the area that is injured. Use a sling, crutches, or splint as needed.

- **Ice**: Apply ice wrapped in a thin towel for 20 minutes every hour to reduce swelling. Do no place the ice directly on the skin.

- **Compression**: Gently wrap the injured joint or limb with an elastic bandage or sleeve to help control swelling. Specialized braces may be more effective for certain injuries.

- **Elevation**: Whenever possible, elevate the injured area above heart level to further reduce swelling.

2. Use over-the-counter pain relievers like ibuprofen (Advil, Motrin), acetaminophen (Tylenol), or aspirin (not for individuals under age 16) to relieve pain and reduce inflammation.

3. For all but the most minor strains and sprains, it's essential to seek evaluation from a doctor.

Consult a medical professional promptly if you observe any of the following symptoms that could indicate a possible broken bone:

- A "popping" sound accompanies the injury.

- The person is unable to move the injured joint or limb or bear weight on it.

- The limb gives way or buckles when the injured joint is used.

- Numbness is present.

- If significant swelling, pain, fever, or open cuts are observed.

4. Continue the RICE (Rest, Ice, Compression, Elevation) method for 24 to 48 hours, or until the person is able to see a doctor. The doctor may recommend X-rays or an MRI to diagnose a severe sprain or strain or to rule out a fracture. Immobilization of the limb or joint may be necessary using a splint, cast, or other device until complete healing occurs. Physical therapy is often beneficial to restore normal function to an injured joint. Surgical procedure may be required in very severe cases.

Signs to Watch For:

- The individual experiences pain or tenderness near the injury site.

- Difficulty moving or putting weight on the injured area.

- Noticeable swelling around the injury.

- Changes in skin color, indicating bruising is starting to appear.

Dealing with Splinters and Blisters

Splinters

A splinter is a small, thin, often sharp fragment of a foreign object that becomes embedded in the skin, typically causing discomfort or pain. Splinters commonly occur when handling wood, metal, or glass objects, and they can lodge themselves beneath the skin's surface. Splinters may cause irritation, inflammation, and sometimes infection if not properly removed and treated.

First Aid for Splinters

1. Start by thoroughly washing your hands and cleaning the affected area with soap and water.

2. Sterilize tweezers using rubbing alcohol before using them to remove the object. For better visibility, consider using a magnifying glass.

3. If the object is embedded under the skin, take a clean, sharp needle and sterilize it with rubbing alcohol. Carefully puncture the skin above the object with the needle to expose its tip.

4. Use the tweezers to grasp the exposed end of the object and gently pull it out.

5. Clean the area again and pat it dry gently. Apply a thin layer of petroleum jelly or antibiotic ointment to the site.

When to Seek Medical Attention

If you encounter a foreign object deeply embedded in the skin or muscle, it's important to seek immediate medical assistance. Follow these steps before getting help:

1. Refrain from trying to remove the object yourself to avoid worsening the situation.

2. Place gauze directly over the object and add clean padding around it if needed. Securely wrap the wound with a bandage or clean cloth, taking care not to apply excessive pressure on the object.

Seek medical attention especially if:

1. The object is hard to see (like clear glass) or difficult to remove (such as a fishhook).

2. The injury is near or involves an eye.

3. The wound is deep or contaminated, and the injured person has not had a tetanus shot in the last five years. In such cases, a tetanus booster may be recommended by a doctor.

Blisters

A blister is a small, fluid-filled bubble that forms on the outer layer of the skin. It typically develops in response to friction, burns, or other types of irritation. The fluid inside a blister is usually clear or slightly yellowish and acts as a protective cushion for the underlying skin. Blisters can be painful or tender and may appear red or swollen around the affected area. They are a natural defense mechanism of the body to protect the skin and aid in the healing process.

Causes of Blisters

The most frequent blisters arise from prolonged friction between the skin and clothing or gear. However, blisters can result from various factors:

1. Wearing shoes without socks or with ill-fitting, low-quality socks.

2. Continued rubbing while gripping sports equipment like tennis racquets, cricket bats, golf clubs, or hockey sticks, as well as gardening or hand tools such as rakes, shovels, picks, hammers, and saws.

3. Exposure to steam, heat, chemicals, or sunburn.

4. Allergic reactions to irritating substances.

Signs and Symptoms

After a blister has formed, you can recognize it by observing the following signs and symptoms:

- A raised bump containing clear fluid or blood
- Redness, tenderness, or itching in the surrounding skin area

First Aid for Blisters

Here are 7 steps for treating blisters effectively:

1. Wear clean medical gloves to reduce the risk of infection.

2. Clean the blister area gently with saline solution.

3. Use a sterile pin to puncture the edge of the blister at 2 or 3 points.

4. Carefully drain the fluid without damaging the skin surface of the blister.

5. Cover the blister with a non-adhesive gauze pad.

6. Secure the dressing with padding and tape.

7. Monitor the area for signs of increased irritation, redness, warmth, or pain. Seek medical attention if these symptoms worsen.

Seeking Medical Assistance for Blisters: Blisters can result from various activities and may lead to complications if not managed promptly or if caused by severe conditions. After providing initial first aid for blisters, it's important to seek medical help if you notice any of these signs:

- The blister is caused by a burn, scald, or severe sunburn.

- The blister starts oozing pus that is yellow or green, or emits an unusual odor.

- The affected area becomes swollen or inflamed.

- You suspect the blister might be infected.

Prevention

To prevent blisters, consider the following measures:

- Wear moisture-wicking or sports socks to reduce friction and rubbing.

- Change wet socks promptly to minimize skin friction.

- Apply tape to areas that show signs of rubbing and tenderness.

- Use sturdy work gloves when handling tools like shovels, rakes, brooms, and hammers.

- Protect yourself from sunburn blisters by wearing sun-protective clothing, hats, and sunscreen with an SPF of 30 or higher.

- Exercise caution around steam, flames, and hot objects.

- Avoid direct contact with chemicals.

Nosebleeds

A nosebleed occurs when a blood vessel in the lining of the nose bursts. This can be triggered by various factors such as infection, injury, allergies, nose picking, or inserting objects into the nostril. Another term for a nosebleed is **Epistaxis**. Nosebleeds are a common occurrence in children and are typically not a cause for concern. However, it's advisable to seek medical attention if nosebleeds are severe, happen frequently, or last for an extended period.

The delicate blood vessels within the septum (the sturdy tissue dividing the nose into two halves) can easily rupture, leading to a nosebleed. In children, nosebleeds typically occur from one side (unilaterally) and often resolve as they grow older. However, if the bleeding is severe, prolonged, or doesn't stop after basic first aid, it's important to seek medical attention promptly. Take your child to a doctor or the emergency department of a hospital for further evaluation and treatment.

Symptoms of Nosebleeds

Common signs and symptoms of a nosebleed may include:

- Blood coming from one or both nostrils

- Feeling of liquid moving down the back of the throat

- Frequent urge to swallow

Causes of Nosebleeds

Here are the various factors that can contribute to nosebleeds:

- Fragile blood vessels that are more prone to bleeding, especially in warm, dry air or after physical exercise.
- Infections affecting the nose lining, sinuses, or adenoids.
- Allergies that trigger hay fever or persistent coughing.
- Trauma from bumps or falls.
- Insertion of foreign objects into the nostril.
- Nose picking.
- In rare cases, underlying bleeding or clotting disorders.

First Aid for Nosebleeds

- Comfort the individual, especially children, to calm them and reduce anxiety, as crying can increase blood flow.
- Seat the person upright and tilt their head slightly forward to prevent blood from flowing backward into the throat.
- Using your finger and thumb, firmly pinch the soft part of the nostrils just below the bridge of the nose. Maintain pressure for at least 10 minutes while the person breathes through their mouth.
- Loosen any tight clothing around the neck and apply a cold cloth or cold pack to the forehead and neck (sides) to help constrict blood vessels.

- After 10 minutes of continuous pressure, release and check if the bleeding has stopped. If the bleeding persists, seek medical attention immediately.

- Advise the person not to sniff or blow their nose for at least 15 minutes to allow a stable clot to form. Avoid nose picking for the remainder of the day to prevent dislodging the clot.

- If bleeding continues despite initial first aid measures, promptly seek medical evaluation to identify and address the underlying cause of the nosebleed.

Basic Burn Care

Burns occur when tissues are damaged due to exposure to heat, sun radiation, chemicals, or electricity. They can range from minor issues to serious emergencies. Treatment for burns varies based on their location and severity. Minor burns like sunburns or small scalds can often be managed with first aid. However, deep or extensive burns require urgent medical attention. Certain cases may necessitate treatment at specialized burn centers and ongoing care over several months.

Burn symptoms can vary depending on the depth of the skin damage. It may take a day or two for signs and symptoms of a severe burn to fully develop.

- First-degree burn: This minor burn affects only the outer layer of the skin (epidermis), causing redness and pain.

- Second-degree burn: This category of burn impacts both the outer layer of skin, known as the epidermis, and the deeper second layer, called the dermis. It can lead to swelling and red, white, or splotchy skin. Blisters may form, and pain can be intense. Deep second-degree burns can result in scarring.

- Third-degree burn: These burns extend through the skin to the fat layer beneath. Affected areas may appear black, brown, or white, with a leathery texture. Third-degree burns can damage nerves, leading to numbness.

First Aid for Minor First-Degree Burns

1. Hold the affected area under cool (not cold) running water or immerse it in cool water until the pain lessens. If running water isn't available, use cool compresses.

2. Cover the burn with a sterile, non-adhesive bandage or clean cloth. Avoid applying butter, oil, lotions, or fragranced creams. Instead, use a petroleum-based ointment two to three times daily.

3. Administer over-the-counter pain relievers like acetaminophen (e.g., Panadol, Tylenol), ibuprofen (e.g., Advil, Motrin), or naproxen (e.g., Aleve, Naprosyn).

4. Consult a doctor if you notice signs of infection such as increased pain, redness, swelling, fever, or oozing. Seek medical attention for a tetanus booster if it's been more than 10 years since the last shot. Visit a healthcare provider if the burn blister exceeds two inches in diameter, oozes, or if redness and pain persist beyond a few hours. Medical evaluation is crucial if the burn affects sensitive areas like the hands, feet, face, or genitals.

5. Visit a doctor for examination and potential prescription of antibiotics or pain medication, if necessary.

First Aid for Second-Degree Burns:

1. Place the affected area under cool running water for 10-15 minutes. Use cool compresses If running water is not readily available. Avoid using ice, as it can worsen pain and damage the skin. Do not pop blisters or apply butter or ointments, as this can lead to infection.

2. Cover the burn loosely with a sterile, nonstick bandage. Secure the bandage in place with gauze or tape to prevent further irritation.

3. Lay the person flat, unless they have a head, neck, or leg injury, or if lying flat causes discomfort. Elevate the feet about 12 inches to help prevent shock. If possible, elevate the burn area above the level of the heart. Ensure to keep the person warm by covering them with a coat or blanket.

4. Visit a doctor to assess the severity of the burn. The doctor may prescribe antibiotics and pain medications. If needed, a tetanus shot may be given.

First Aid for Severe (Third-Degree) Burns:

1. Call 911 immediately.

2. Gently cover the burn with a sterile, nonstick bandage or a clean, lint-free material to prevent infection. If fingers or toes are affected, use dry, sterile dressings to separate them. Avoid soaking the burn in water or applying ointments or butter, as these can lead to infection.

3. Lay the person flat, unless they have a head, neck, or leg injury, or if lying flat is uncomfortable. Elevate the feet by about 12 inches. If feasible, raise the burned area so that it is positioned higher than the heart. Cover the person with a coat or blanket for warmth. Do not use a pillow under the head if there's an airway burn, as this can obstruct breathing. If the person has a facial burn, have them sit up. Continuously monitor pulse and breathing for signs of shock until emergency help arrives.

4. It's crucial to seek medical help promptly. Doctors will administer oxygen and fluids as needed and provide appropriate treatment for the burn.

CHAPTER 5: ADDRESSING COMMON ILLNESSES

This chapter explores practical strategies for managing everyday illnesses that can affect individuals of all ages. From the common cold to stomach upset, understanding how to recognize symptoms and provide appropriate care is essential for maintaining well-being. By empowering readers with the knowledge to address these illnesses promptly and effectively, this chapter aims to promote proactive health management and enhance overall comfort during times of minor illness.

Recognizing and Managing Earache

An earache, also known as **Otalgia**, is a common symptom characterized by pain or discomfort in the ear. It can affect individuals of all ages and may vary in severity and duration. Ear pain may arise from a variety of causes, such as:

1. Ear Infections: One of the most common causes of earaches is middle ear infections (otitis media), particularly in children. These infections often result from bacterial or viral infections, leading to inflammation and fluid buildup behind the eardrum.

2. Outer Ear Infections: Infections of the external ear canal (otitis externa or swimmer's ear) can cause earaches. These infections are often associated with exposure to water, which creates a favorable environment for bacterial or fungal growth.

3. Blockages: Earwax buildup or foreign objects lodged in the ear can cause pressure and discomfort, leading to earaches.

4. Trauma or Injury: Injury to the ear, such as from a blow to the ear or insertion of objects into the ear canal, can result in pain and earaches.

5. Allergies or Sinusitis: Conditions affecting the upper respiratory tract, such as allergies or sinus infections, can sometimes lead to referred pain in the ears.

Symptoms of an earache can vary but often include:

- Sharp or dull pain in the ear

- Feeling pressure or fullness in the ear

- Tenderness around the ear

- Itching or irritation

- Hearing loss or changes in hearing

- Fever (especially in the case of infections)

First Aid for Earache

An earache can be a painful and uncomfortable experience. While waiting for medical attention, there are several steps you can take to provide relief:

➢ Determine the severity of the earache and look for any other symptoms such as fever or discharge from the ear.

➢ Offer over-the-counter pain relievers like acetaminophen (Tylenol) or ibuprofen (Advil) to help reduce pain and inflammation. Follow dosage instructions based on age and medical history.

➢ Place a warm, moist washcloth or heating pad against the affected ear. The warmth can help soothe the pain and reduce tension in the ear canal.

➢ Avoid getting water or any other fluids into the ear. Moisture can worsen the pain and potentially lead to infection.

➢ Encourage the person to rest in a comfortable position with the affected ear elevated. This can help in alleviating the pressure and discomfort.

➢ Advise against inserting cotton swabs or other objects into the ear canal. This can push debris further inside or cause injury.

➢ Be at alert for some of the symptoms and note any changes. If there's persistent pain, fever, or worsening of symptoms, seek medical attention promptly.

➢ It's important to consult a healthcare professional if the earache persists or if there are additional symptoms like ear discharge, hearing loss, or dizziness.

Coping with Diarrhea

Most cases of diarrhea, characterized by loose or watery bowel movements, are often caused by a viral infection in the intestines. While diarrhea is typically not a sign of a serious illness, it can lead to dehydration and loss of essential fluids, salts, and minerals in both children and adults. Therefore, it's important to ensure that fluids and nutrients are replenished when experiencing diarrhea, regardless of age.

Signs & Symptoms of Diarrhea

- Loose and frequent bowel movements (poops)

- Cramping or belly pain

- Fever

- Loss of appetite

- Feeling tired or fatigued

- Unintended weight loss

- Dehydration

First Aid for Diarrhea

When experiencing mild diarrhea, it can often be managed effectively with simple remedies. Here's how you can address diarrhea symptoms:

1. Drink plenty of water and electrolyte-balanced fluids like sports drinks, broths, diluted fruit juices, and caffeine-free sodas to replace lost fluids and electrolytes.

2. Opt for low-fiber foods like those in the BRAT diet—bananas, white rice, applesauce, and toast. Other suitable options include lean meats, noodles, potatoes, and skinless turkey, chicken, or fish.

3. Steer clear of carbonated beverages, Brussels sprouts, beer, cabbage, and beans, as they can cause stomach discomfort. Temporarily avoid dairy products if diarrhea has made you lactose intolerant.

4. Alcohol can dehydrate you, while caffeinated drinks can worsen diarrhea due to their mild laxative effect. Avoid chocolate, green tea, strong tea, sodas, and coffee.

5. Over-the-counter options like loperamide and bismuth subsalicylate can help control symptoms and reduce watery stools. Always consult your doctor before using these medications, especially for children.

6. Probiotics can restore healthy gut bacteria. Consult your doctor before starting probiotics, available in liquid or capsule form and sometimes added to certain foods.

When to Consult a Doctor for Diarrhea:

If you have diarrhea, it's important to reach out to your doctor in the following situations:

- If your diarrhea has lasted for more than two days.
- If you notice stains of blood in your stools or if your stools appear black.
- If you have a fever above 39 degrees Celsius (102 degrees Fahrenheit).
- If you experience intense pain in your abdomen or rectum.
- If you feel dehydrated, indicated by thirst, dry mouth, or decreased urination.
- If you are unable to drink fluids due to persistent nausea or vomiting.
- If you develop diarrhea after returning from a foreign destination.

Managing Cold

Cooling of body parts can lead to various cold-related injuries, with hypothermia being the most serious. Nonfreezing cold injuries include chilblain, immersion foot, and trench foot, while freezing injuries encompass windburn, frostnip, and frostbite. Body parts such as toes, fingers, ears, and nose are particularly vulnerable due to the lack of major muscles to generate heat. The body conserves heat by reducing blood flow to these extremities in cold conditions. Additionally, hands and feet cool faster than the torso because they have a higher surface area-to-volume ratio and are more likely to come into contact with cold surfaces.

Exposure of the eyes to high wind chill without protection (like goggles) can lead to freezing of the corneas. Hypothermia, characterized by excessive loss of body heat and a drop in core temperature, is the most severe cold injury and can be life-threatening.

Taking immediate action can prevent further heat loss and gradually warm up the body.

1. Stay calm to avoid excessive sweating, which can make you feel colder.

2. Seek shelter from the cold, wind, or water.

3. Remove wet clothing and replace it with dry clothing, preferably wool or synthetic fabrics that provide good insulation. Cover your head.

4. If dry clothing is unavailable, try skin-to-skin contact with another person under a blanket or sleeping bag to share body heat.

5. Use a heated blanket if accessible.

6. Engage in light movement to boost blood flow and body heat without sweating excessively.

7. Drink warm fluids (avoid caffeine or alcohol) and eat high-energy foods like candy. Avoid giving food or drink to confused or slow-responding individuals.

8. Avoid full-body immersion in warm water unless absolutely necessary. Instead, warm small body parts like hands or feet in warm water (38°C to 41°C).

9. Avoid tobacco, as it can worsen circulation.

10. Be cautious near heat sources to prevent burns, as cold-injured skin may not feel heat normally.

For frostbite or cold-exposed body parts:

- Protect the affected area to avoid further exposure to cold.

- Do not rub or massage the skin if frozen.

- Avoid rewarming if refreezing is possible; seek shelter first.

- Use gentle warming methods like blowing warm air onto cold hands or using warm water (40°C to 42°C) for localized thawing.

- Pad and wrap frozen fingers or toes in soft, dry material to prevent further damage.

Understanding Hypothermia

Hypothermia occurs when the body's core temperature drops significantly due to prolonged exposure to cold conditions, especially without adequate protection. Normally, the body can adapt to moderately cold environments by maintaining its core temperature close to 37°C (98.6°F). However, in extreme cold or when exposed for too long without proper clothing, the body's heat loss exceeds its ability to generate warmth.

The early signs of mild hypothermia include feeling cold and experiencing pain in exposed areas of the body. As the temperature continues to decrease or exposure time lengthens, the sensation of cold and pain diminishes due to numbness, making it difficult for the person to recognize serious injury. Muscular weakness, drowsiness, and interrupted shivering may follow, accompanied by diminished consciousness and dilated pupils. Severe hypothermia can lead to life-threatening symptoms, including death, if not promptly treated.

What are the signs of hypothermia?

The Red Cross identifies different levels of cold stress, including:

Cold stress (not hypothermic):

- Shivering
- Normal mental status
- Able to care for oneself

Mild hypothermia:

- Vigorous shivering and complaints of feeling cold
- Decreased physical function
- Difficulty taking care of oneself

Moderate hypothermia:

- Weak or intermittent shivering, possibly ceasing later
- Occasional complaints of feeling cold
- Lack of coordination or speech; confusion or unusual behavior
- Impaired judgment
- Potential unresponsiveness

Severe hypothermia:

- Cessation of shivering

- Unresponsiveness; slowed or stopped breathing
- Stiff body
- Absence of pulse

First Aid for Hypothermia

Hypothermia is a serious medical emergency that requires immediate medical attention. It's crucial to act swiftly and appropriately to prevent further complications and aid in the victim's recovery.

- ➢ Call for medical assistance immediately upon recognizing signs of hypothermia. Timing is crucial when addressing this condition.
- ➢ The person out of the cold environment and into a warmer place. Insulate them from the cold ground or surroundings.
- ➢ Check the person's (ABCs) airway, breathing, and circulation. If necessary, administer CPR.
- ➢ Avoid massaging or rubbing the person's skin, as this can cause further damage.
- ➢ Lay the person down gently. Avoid standing or walking, as movement can worsen the condition.
- ➢ Use warm water bottles, heating pads, or electric blankets to warm specific areas like the armpits, chest, groin, and upper back. Wrap these items in towels or clothing to prevent direct contact with the skin. If available, use body heat from another person to help warm the victim.
- ➢ Do not use direct heat sources like heating lamps, stoves, hot baths, or showers for rewarming, as this can be harmful.
- ➢ Offer caffeine-free, non-alcoholic drinks only if the person is conscious and responsive. Avoid giving food or fluids if the person is severely hypothermic or unconscious.
- ➢ If the person stops breathing or shows no signs of circulation, administer CPR until medical help arrives. In some cases, hypothermia victims who appear unconscious or "dead" have been successfully resuscitated.

Headaches

Experiencing a sleepless night, skipping meals, dealing with a tooth infection, or recovering from a hangover—these are just a few reasons why people might get a headache. While some find relief in a cup of tea or a nap, the true nature of headaches is far more complex.

A headache refers to pain perceived in any part of the head. Despite its common occurrence, it's crucial not to dismiss this symptom. Frequent headaches have been associated with various serious medical conditions. Therefore, it's important to consult a doctor to understand the underlying cause of your headaches and receive appropriate treatment to alleviate them effectively.

Types of Headaches

Did you know that the International Headache Society classifies over 150 types of headaches? When you consult a doctor for a headache, they typically inquire about specific details to help diagnose the issue:

- Where is the pain located?

- How did the headache start? Was it sudden and sharp or more gradual?

- How long does the headache typically last?

- Are there any accompanying symptoms?

- What activities or factors worsen or alleviate the pain?

Gathering these details assists doctors in pinpointing the potential cause of the headache.

Headaches are generally categorized as follows:

Primary Headaches: These stem from pain-sensitive structures in the head, excluding the brain itself, which lacks pain receptors. Pain-sensitive areas like blood vessels, muscles, meninges (brain covering), eyes, ears, or teeth can be triggered by various factors.

Secondary Headaches: When a headache results from an underlying disorder or condition, it falls into the secondary headache category. Many diseases can cause headaches, often accompanied by specific indicative symptoms.

Primary Headaches

The most prevalent primary headaches include migraines, cluster headaches, and tension headaches, affecting approximately 90% of headache sufferers. Migraines typically involve intense throbbing pain, often worsened by light and sound, accompanied by nausea and sometimes preceded by visual disturbances known as aura. Tension headaches are characterized by a sensation of pressure around the head, usually without throbbing pain or additional symptoms. Cluster headaches manifest as brief, intense pain localized around one eye, often accompanied by nasal congestion, eye redness, and increased tear production, typically occurring at consistent daily intervals.

Various lifestyle factors can contribute to frequent primary headaches, including:

- Alcohol consumption
- High stress levels
- Inadequate sleep
- Poor posture
- Skipping meals
- Consumption of certain foods containing nitrates (e.g., aged cheese)
- Headaches triggered by physical exertion or exercise
- "Brain freeze" headaches caused by consuming very cold items

Secondary headaches

Secondary headaches are symptoms caused by an underlying disease or condition. Common contributors to secondary headaches include:

- Sinusitis
- Ear infection
- Tooth infection

- Generalized infections like flu

- Dehydration

- Side effects of medications

- Head trauma or concussions

- Meningitis (infection of the meninges)

- Encephalitis (infection of brain tissue)

- High blood pressure (hypertension)

- Stroke

- Intracranial bleeding

- Hemorrhages and blood vessel issues

- Glaucoma (increased pressure inside the eyeball)

These headaches are distinct from primary headaches, which are not caused by an underlying condition but rather by overactivity or problems with pain-sensitive structures in the head.

First aid for Headache

As we spend extended hours glued to screens, experience irregular sleep patterns, and often neglect hydration, headaches have become increasingly common. Here are some immediate measures you can take at home to alleviate your headache:

- Reduce exposure to triggers such as bright lights, loud noises, screen use (TV, phone), and strong fragrances, all of which can provoke headaches in some individuals.

- Rest is crucial for managing headaches. Find a relatively cool, dark, and quiet room to relax in.

- Adequate sleep is essential for reducing headache severity. Applying cold compresses or ice packs to your forehead may offer temporary relief.

- Over-the-counter pain medications like Paracetamol (acetaminophen) are readily available and safe for managing headaches. Adults can take a dose of 500-1000mg up to three times a day. Remember to eat and drink before taking medication.

- Stress management and relaxation techniques can help desensitize you and prevent stress-induced headaches.

- Acupuncture has demonstrated effectiveness in relieving chronic headaches such as migraines.

Frequent headaches with other symptoms warrant a doctor's visit to identify and address the underlying cause. Ensure to Seek immediate medical attention if you experience the following:

- A sudden, extremely severe headache.
- Headaches that worsen rapidly over hours or days.
- Changes in mental alertness, consciousness, or perception.
- Seizures or loss of consciousness.
- Experiencing a new types of headaches after age 50.
- Personality changes or abnormal behavior.
- Recent head injury.
- Headaches accompanied by:
  - Fever.
  - Stiff neck.
  - Vomiting.
  - Severe eye pain.
  - Weakness or paralysis in limbs.
  - Difficulty walking or using hands.
  - Slurred speech.
  - Loss of balance.
  - Double vision, seeing colored halos, or sudden vision loss.

These symptoms suggest serious underlying causes that require prompt medical evaluation and treatment.

Handling Motion Sickness

Are you someone who loves to travel but dreads getting into a car because it makes you feel nauseated? Does the idea of riding a roller coaster make your stomach churn? If you answered yes to these questions, you may be experiencing motion sickness (MS). In this section, we'll provide an overview of motion sickness, along with helpful tips for preventing and reducing its effects so you can enjoy your travels without discomfort.

Common Signs and Symptoms of Motion Sickness:

- Sweating

- Feeling tired or fatigued

- Paleness or a pale complexion

- Nausea

- Vomiting

- Dizziness or feeling lightheaded

- Increased saliva production

- Abdominal discomfort or uneasiness in the stomach

- Headache

- Loss of appetite

- Blurred vision

- Ringing sensation in the ears (tinnitus)

- Cold and clammy skin

Causes of Motion Sickness

Motion sickness commonly occurs due to a discrepancy between the visual cues and signals from the vestibular system, which controls balance and spatial orientation.

When you're in a moving vehicle or on a platform, your eyes perceive motion and changes in direction, but your vestibular system doesn't register these changes. This mismatch between sensory inputs leads to feelings of disorientation and dizziness, characteristic of motion sickness.

Additionally, other factors can contribute to motion sickness, such as low blood sugar levels, anxiety, fatigue, and certain medications. Lack of sufficient sleep or exposure to strong odors in the vehicle can also increase susceptibility to motion sickness. Interestingly, for some individuals, merely anticipating motion can be enough to trigger symptoms of motion sickness.

Types of Motion Sickness

Motion sickness can manifest in various forms depending on the environment or activity. Here are the common types:

1. **Seasickness**: Occurs on boats due to the rocking motion combined with visual cues like the horizon or waves. Symptoms include dizziness, nausea, vomiting, and sweating.

2. **Airsickness**: Experienced during flights at high altitudes due to turbulence, leading to nausea and possibly vomiting.

3. **Car Sickness**: Happens during car rides or amusement park trips, triggered by vehicle motion or environmental factors. Symptoms may include nausea and vomiting.

4. **Ride Sickness**: Caused by abrupt and jerky movements on amusement park rides, resulting in dizziness and potential vomiting.

5. **Virtual Reality Sickness**: Occurs when using a virtual reality headset, causing sensations of nausea and dizziness due to the immersive 3D environment.

First aid for Motion Sickness

Here's a practical guide for managing motion sickness:

1. Sit upright in the car, bus, or boat; avoid lying down.

2. Focus on the horizon or a distant object to stabilize your gaze.

3. Take slow, deep breaths to help calm your stomach.

4. Request your travel companion to drive smoothly and avoid sudden movements.

5. Refrain from reading or using your phone to minimize visual stimulation.

6. Avoid consuming fatty or greasy foods before and during travel.

7. If prescribed by your doctor, consider taking medications like dimenhydrinate (Dramamine) or meclizine (Bonine).

8. Consume ginger in various forms such as ginger candy or ginger ale, known for its anti-nausea properties.

9. Try sipping lemonade or sucking on a lemon wedge to increase saliva production, which can ease nausea sensations.

Self-Care Tips for Traveling

Here are some effective measures you can take to reduce motion sickness while traveling:

- Practice rest and relaxation techniques like deep breathing and visualization during your journey.
- Take frequent breaks from traveling to alleviate symptoms.
- Stay hydrated by increasing fluid intake and avoiding alcohol.
- Opt for light, non-heavy meals that are gentle on the stomach.
- Eat small meals throughout the day to help manage nausea.
- Ensure you get plenty of rest before embarking on your journey.
- Avoid consuming fatty or spicy foods, which can exacerbate symptoms.
- Refrain from reading or watching TV while in transit.
- Listen to calming music or use earplugs to minimize visual stimulation.
- Consider using motion sickness prevention methods such as antihistamines or acupuncture before traveling.
- Open a window for fresh air, which can help alleviate nausea.
- Choose a seat that faces the direction of travel to reduce motion sickness.

Panic Attacks

Approximately six million adults in the United States have panic disorder, a condition characterized by recurring episodes of intense fear known as panic attacks. Furthermore, panic attacks can occur in individuals without a diagnosed panic disorder. In fact, more than one in five people will experience a panic attack at some point in their lives. Do you know what to do if you encounter someone having a panic attack? If not, don't worry. This section will explain how to assist someone experiencing a panic attack, ensuring you feel prepared to offer help when needed.

How to recognize a Panic Attack

To identify whether someone is experiencing a panic attack due to fear, anxiety, or a physical cause, it's essential to recognize specific symptoms. Here are ten common signs of a panic attack to watch for:

- Feeling shaky

- Experiencing sweating

- Numbness or tingling sensations

- Feeling dizzy

- Chest pain or discomfort

- Abdominal distress (such as stomach pain, nausea, or indigestion)

- Fear of losing control, experiencing a sense of insanity, or facing mortality

- Chills or hot flashes (sudden sensations of heat or cold)

- Heart palpitations, characterized by the sensation of your heart racing or pounding

- Difficulty breathing or sensation of inadequate air intake.

Supporting Someone During a Panic Attack

If you suspect someone is experiencing a panic attack, follow the **ALGEE** steps recommended by Mental Health First Aid:

> **Assess for Risk**: Inquire if they have experienced this before and if they believe they are having one now. If they confirm and want assistance, introduce yourself if they are a stranger.

> **Listen Without Judgment**: Directly ask what they think might help, such as moving to a quieter area or sitting down. Avoid assuming you know the best solution for them.

> **Provide Reassurance and Information**: Stay calm and reassure them that they are likely having a panic attack, which is not harmful. Explain that while it's scary, the symptoms will subside. Speak in short, clear sentences with a firm tone. Be patient and remain with them until the attack passes.

> **Encourage seeking appropriate professional support**: After the panic attack subsides, offer the individual information about panic attacks if they are unfamiliar or unsure where to find resources. If they express worry, assure them that effective treatments exist for panic attacks and emphasize that help is accessible to them.

CHAPTER 6: RESPONDING TO TRAUMATIC INJURIES

Encountering traumatic injuries can be daunting, but having the knowledge and skills to respond effectively can make a life-saving difference. This chapter is designed to equip you with essential techniques and strategies for managing traumatic incidents with confidence and competence.

From serious wounds and fractures to head injuries and critical emergencies, traumatic injuries demand swift and appropriate action. Whether you're a professional responder or a concerned bystander, understanding how to assess, stabilize, and provide initial care is crucial. Throughout this chapter, we'll explore key principles including scene safety assessment, basic life support measures, fracture stabilization, head and spinal injury management, and shock recognition and treatment.

Managing Severe Bleeding

Bleeding occurs when blood exits the circulatory system, often due to cuts, abrasions, or more serious injuries like deep cuts or amputations. Internal bleeding, caused by trauma to the body, can also occur and may range from minor (resulting in superficial bruising) to severe hemorrhaging.

Providing prompt first aid for severe external or internal bleeding is crucial to minimize blood loss until professional medical assistance arrives. Immediate actions for managing external bleeding involve applying direct pressure to the wound, maintaining pressure using pads and bandages, and elevating the injured limb above the level of the heart if feasible. These steps help control bleeding and stabilize the injured person's condition until further medical treatment can be administered.

First Aid For Severe Bleeding

In the event of severe bleeding, it's crucial to take these steps:

1. Begin by putting on disposable gloves and any available personal protective equipment before assessing the wound.

2. Carefully remove any clothing or debris from the wound to locate the source of bleeding. Avoid attempting to clean the wound at this stage.

3. Once identified, apply firm pressure to the wound using sterile gauze or a clean cloth. Use your palm to press down firmly until the bleeding stops.

4. Securely wrap the wound with a thick bandage and tape. If possible, elevate the wound above heart level to reduce blood flow.

5. Help the injured person lie down on a rug or blanket to maintain body heat. If signs of shock (weakness, clammy skin, rapid pulse) are observed, elevate their feet.

6. Reassure the injured person and continue to monitor their condition closely.

7. Apply additional bandages if blood seeps through, maintaining firm pressure on the area.

8. Use a tourniquet only as a last resort for life-threatening bleeding on a limb, and apply it correctly if trained. Remember to note the time it was applied.

9. Keep the injured person still and wait for emergency help if needed. If help hasn't been called, transport the injured person to an emergency room promptly.

10. Remember to wash your hands thoroughly after providing aid, regardless of blood exposure.

Here are important precautions to follow when providing first aid:

- Avoid removing large or deeply embedded objects from a wound.
- Refrain from probing or digging into the wound.
- Do not apply pressure to an eye injury or an embedded object near the eye.
- Avoid pressing wounds on the head if you suspect a skull fracture.
- Do not use improvised tourniquets, such as scarves or belts, as they may not effectively control bleeding and could cause further harm.

Amputation

Amputation involves the removal of a body part, which can occur in a hospital setting under medical supervision or as a result of an accident or mishap. Amputations can be categorized as complete, where the body part is entirely severed, or partial, where a significant portion of the body part is removed but remains attached. Reattachment of amputated parts is possible in some cases. The success of reattachment depends on several factors:

- The specific body part involved in the amputation.

- The condition of the amputated part (how well it was preserved).

- The time elapsed between the amputation and receiving medical care.

- The overall health and condition of the injured individual.

Successful reattachment requires prompt medical attention and favorable circumstances related to the amputated part and the person's health.

Here are the steps to assist someone who has experienced an accidental amputation:

1. Immediately call emergency services for urgent medical assistance.

2. Although complete amputations may not bleed significantly due to blood vessel spasms, take these steps if bleeding occurs:

   - If available, wash your hands with soap and water and wear disposable gloves.

   - If gloves are unavailable, use multiple layers of clean cloth, plastic bags, or the cleanest material accessible to apply pressure on the wound.

   - Instruct the injured person lie down and elevate the bleeding site.

   - Remove any visible objects from the wound and cut away clothing around the injury.

   - Apply steady direct pressure on the wound for a full 15 minutes.

   - If bleeding persists or is severe, continue applying pressure while seeking assistance.

3. If the amputated part is recovered:

   - Gently rinse off dirt and debris with clean water (do not scrub).

   - Wrap the amputated part in a dry, sterile gauze.

- Place the wrapped part in a plastic bag or waterproof container.

- Keep the amputated part cool by placing the bag/container on ice (avoid direct contact with ice or ice water).

4. Transport both the injured person and the amputated part to the hospital as quickly as possible. If the severed part cannot be promptly located, focus on transporting the injured individual to the hospital first and bring the amputated part with you once it is found.

If a body part has been partially amputated, follow these steps:

- Elevate the injured area to help reduce blood flow and swelling.
- Cover the injured area with a sterile dressing or clean cloth to protect it.
- Apply light pressure if there is bleeding to help slow it down, but avoid cutting off blood flow to the amputated part.
- Use a gentle splint to immobilize the injured area and prevent further damage or movement.

Shock

Shock is a serious condition caused by a sudden decrease in blood flow throughout the body. It can be triggered by various factors such as trauma, heatstroke, blood loss, allergic reactions, severe infection, poisoning, or severe burns. In shock, vital organs do not receive adequate blood supply or oxygen, which can lead to permanent organ damage or death if left untreated. Therefore, prompt recognition and appropriate treatment are essential to prevent serious consequences.

When to Seek Emergency Care:

If you suspect that a person is experiencing shock, it's important to call 911 or your local emergency number immediately.

Symptoms of Shock:

Symptoms of shock can vary depending on the situation and may include:

- Cool, clammy skin

- Pale or ashen skin

- Bluish or grayish lips or fingernails

- Rapid pulse

- Fast breathing

- Nausea or vomiting

- Dilated (enlarged) pupils

- Weakness or fatigue

- Dizziness or fainting

- Alterations in mental condition or demeanor

Causes of Shock

Shock can be caused by various medical conditions, which include:

1. **Low Blood Volume**: This can occur due to severe bleeding (hemorrhage), dehydration, or fluid loss from burns or severe vomiting/diarrhea.

2. **Inadequate Heart Pumping Action**: Conditions such as heart attacks (myocardial infarction), heart failure, or arrhythmias (irregular heartbeats) can impair the heart's ability to pump blood effectively.

3. **Excessive Blood Vessel Dilation**: This can result from severe infections (septic shock), allergic reactions (anaphylactic shock), or neurological injuries that cause blood vessels to dilate uncontrollably.

4. **Medications**: Certain medications that decrease heart function or cause blood vessel dilation can contribute to shock.

5. **Nervous System Damage**: Trauma, spinal cord injuries, or severe brain injuries can disrupt the nervous system's regulation of blood pressure and heart rate, leading to shock.

Types of Shock

The four main types of shock are:

1. **Hypovolemic Shock**: This type of shock occurs due to low blood volume, which leads to insufficient blood being pumped out to the body. Causes include excessive external or internal bleeding, fluid loss from burns or other conditions, severe dehydration, or certain medical disorders affecting fluid balance.

2. **Cardiogenic Shock**: Resulting from heart damage that impairs its ability to pump sufficient blood, cardiogenic shock can stem from conditions such as heart attack, heart valve issues, abnormal heart rhythms, heart muscle infections, or heart valve problems.

3. **Obstructive Shock**: Obstructive shock arises from physical blockages that impede normal blood flow, such as blood clots in the lungs (pulmonary embolism), tension pneumothorax (air trapping in the chest), cardiac tamponade (fluid accumulation around the heart), or other similar obstructions.

4. **Distributive Shock**: This type involves excessive widening (dilation) of blood vessels, which reduces blood pressure and hampers adequate blood flow to organs. Subtypes include:

   - **Anaphylactic Shock**: Usually Caused by severe allergic reactions.

   - **Septic Shock**: Arising from severe bacterial infections in the bloodstream.

   - **Neurogenic Shock**: Resulting from nervous system damage, often due to spinal cord injuries.

   - **Distributive shock:** can also occur due to drug overdoses, brain injuries, or certain endocrine disorders like Addison's disease. Each subtype involves unique mechanisms impacting blood vessel dilation and organ perfusion.

First Aid for Shock

The first aid treatment for shock involves the following steps:

1. Immediately call 911 or your local emergency department to request medical assistance.

2. Assess the person's breathing. If they are not breathing, start rescue breathing and CPR (Cardiopulmonary Resuscitation) if you are trained to do so. If the person is breathing, monitor their breathing every five minutes until help arrives.

3. If the person is conscious and does not have head, neck, spine, or leg injuries, lay them down on their back. Elevate their feet about 12 inches to improve blood flow, but do not elevate their head. If raising their legs could cause pain, lay them flat. Ensure the person is warm and comfortable by covering them with a blanket. Loosen any tight clothing to aid in circulation.

4. If the person has visible wounds and you are trained, provide appropriate first aid to control bleeding. Apply pressure to the wounds using sterile dressings or clean cloth.

5. If the person begins to vomit, drool, or bleed from the mouth (and does not have a spinal injury), turn their head to the side to prevent choking.

6. If you suspect the person has a spinal injury, perform a "log roll":

   a. Keep the person's head, neck, and back in line.

   b. Roll their body and head together as a unit to avoid further injury.

Here are important actions to avoid when providing first aid for shock:

- Refrain from giving the person anything by mouth, including food or drink.
- Avoid moving the person if you suspect they may have a spinal injury.
- Only move the person if they are in immediate danger.
- Do not delay in calling for help, even if the shock symptoms appear mild.

Dislocations

Dislocation occurs when the bones in a joint are forcefully displaced from their normal position. Joints are where two bones meet and are essential components of the skeletal system, providing support and mobility throughout the body.

Dislocations can affect any joint in the body, causing significant pain and impairing joint function. They can also damage surrounding tissues, including muscles, nerves, tendons, and blood vessels. The impact of a dislocation extends beyond the bones, affecting the interconnected structures that facilitate movement and sensation.

When a joint is dislocated, immediate medical attention is often required to realign the bones and address any associated injuries. Proper treatment and rehabilitation are essential to restore joint function and prevent long-term complications. Understanding the risks and symptoms of dislocations can help individuals recognize and respond promptly to these serious injuries.

Types of Dislocation

Dislocations can be classified into different types based on the extent of bone movement in your joints:

1. **Complete Dislocation (Luxation)**: A full dislocation happens when the bones within a joint are fully separated and shifted from their usual alignment.

2. **Subluxation**: Subluxation refers to a partial dislocation where the joint surfaces are partially separated, causing the bones to touch but not in their usual alignment.

Part of The Body Most Prone to Dislocation

Dislocations are relatively common occurrences, with certain joints more prone to this type of injury. The most frequently dislocated joints include:

- Fingers

- Shoulders

- Knees

- Elbows

- Hips

- Jaws

- Collarbone

- Wrist

- Ankle

- Foot

Symptoms of a dislocation typically include:

- Pain
- Swelling
- Bruising
- Noticeable deformity or displacement of the joint
- Inability to move or use the joint
- Sensation of instability or weakness within the joint

The specific symptoms can vary depending on the affected joint and the type of dislocation.

First Aid For Dislocation

Follow these steps for assisting someone with a dislocated joint:

- ➤ **Step 1**: Advise the casualty to remain still and assist them in supporting their dislocated joint in a comfortable position. Avoid attempting to relocate the dislocated bone as this can cause further harm.

- ➤ **Step 2**: Immobilize the joint to prevent movement. If it's a shoulder or elbow dislocation, support the injured arm with a sling. For added stability, use a broad-fold bandage around the chest and sling. If the hand or arm is affected, remove any rings or watches to accommodate swelling. For ankle, knee, or hip dislocations, support the injured leg with padding and broad-fold bandages.

- ➤ **Step 3**: Arrange for the casualty to be taken to the hospital. If you're unable to transport them yourself, call emergency services at 911 for assistance.

- ➤ **Step 4**: While awaiting medical help, attend to shock if necessary by monitoring the casualty's responsiveness. Avoid elevating an injured leg; only raise the uninjured leg if needed.

> **Step 5**: Regularly check circulation beyond any bandages every 10 minutes and adjust or loosen them as required to ensure proper blood flow.

Head Injuries

If you've fallen and hit your head, it's important to assess whether you have a minor head injury or if further attention is needed. Understanding the difference between minor and serious head injuries can be crucial for your well-being. Head injuries are quite common, with millions of people experiencing them each year due to various reasons like accidents, falls, sports activities, or workplace incidents. Fortunately, most head injuries are minor because the skull acts as a natural protective barrier for the brain. However, in some cases, this protection may not be sufficient.

Over half a million people annually require hospitalization due to more severe head injuries. Concussions are the most frequent type of head injury, resulting from a blow that causes the brain to shake within the skull. More serious injuries include brain contusions (bruising of the brain), fractured skulls, or scalp cuts.

It's important to distinguish between **Closed Head Injuries** (where no external bleeding occurs) and **Open Head Injuries** (where an object penetrates the brain, such as glass or a bullet). Understanding these distinctions can aid in recognizing when immediate medical attention is necessary.

Causes of Head Injuries

Head injuries can be attributed to various factors, including:

- Accidents that occur at home, work, during outdoor activities, or while engaging in sports

- Falls

- Physical assaults

- Traffic accidents

Many of these incidents result in minor injuries due to the protective nature of the skull around the brain. However, certain injuries can be severe enough to necessitate hospitalization.

First Aid for Head Injuries

Recognizing and responding to a serious head injury promptly can be life-saving. For a moderate to severe head injury, it's crucial to call 911 or the local emergency number immediately.

Seek immediate medical attention if the injured person experiences any of the following:

- Excessive drowsiness or difficulty staying awake

- Unusual behavior or incoherent speech

- Severe headache or stiff neck

- Seizure activity

- Unequal pupil sizes (anisocoria)

- Inability to move all or part of an arm or leg

- Loss of consciousness, even momentarily

- Persistent vomiting (more than once)

Here are the steps to follow for managing head injuries and suspected spinal injuries:

➤ Check the person's airway, breathing, and circulationCommence rescue breathing and CPR if needed.

➤ If the person is unconscious with normal breathing and heart rate, treat them as if they have a spinal injury. Ensure the head and neck are secure by placing your hands on either side of the head, maintaining alignment with the spine. Prevent any movement and wait for medical assistance.

➤ Stop any bleeding by applying firm pressure with a clean cloth to the wound, unless you suspect a skull fracture. Avoid moving the person's head if the injury is serious. If blood soaks through the cloth, do not remove it; instead, place another cloth over the first one.

➤ If you believe there's a skull fracture, avoid putting direct pressure on the injury or attempting to clear any debris. Instead, use a sterile gauze dressing to cover the wound.

- If the individual is experiencing vomiting or is prone to it, to avoid choking, gently roll their head, neck, and body together onto their side. Maintain stabilization of the head and neck to protect the spine, assuming it is injured in the case of a head injury. Seek further guidance from a healthcare provider.
- Apply ice packs to swollen areas, ensuring to cover the ice with a towel to prevent direct contact with the skin.

Here are important precautions to follow for head injuries:

- Avoid washing a deep or heavily bleeding head wound.
- Do not remove any object protruding from a wound.
- Only move the person if absolutely necessary to avoid exacerbating the injury.
- Refrain from shaking a person who appears dazed.
- Do not remove a helmet if a serious head injury is suspected.
- If a child with signs of head injury has fallen, avoid picking them up.
- Abstain from alcohol or illicit drug use within 48 hours of a serious head injury.
- Seek immediate medical attention for head injuries involving bleeding or suspected brain damage, as they require hospital treatment.
- For mild head injuries, monitor for symptoms and seek medical advice from a healthcare provider. Symptoms of a head injury may manifest later, warranting medical evaluation.

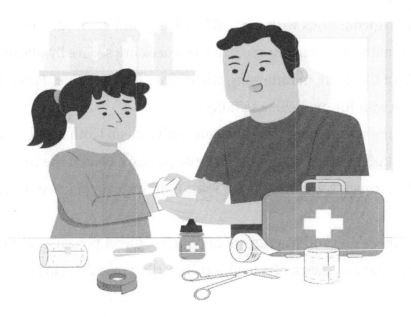

CHAPTER 7: MUSCLE, BONE, AND JOINT INJURIES

Muscle injuries involve strains or tears in muscle fibers, often caused by overexertion or sudden movements. Bone injuries such as fractures can range from simple cracks to complete breaks, requiring immediate attention to prevent further damage. Joint injuries like dislocations and sprains affect the connections between bones, leading to pain and reduced mobility.

By delving into the specifics of muscle, bone, and joint injuries, you'll gain the knowledge needed to recognize these injuries and administer appropriate first aid techniques. Let's explore how to effectively manage and alleviate the discomfort associated with these common injuries.

Shoulder Injuries

Shoulder injuries often affect individuals engaged in sports, weightlifting, or other strenuous activities, leading to significant pain and potential limitations in physical activities. The right treatment and self-care strategies can aid in faster recovery from these injuries.

These injuries can be categorized as acute, occurring suddenly, or chronic, persisting over time. Acute injuries, resulting from falls on outstretched hands or overexertion, are more common than chronic ones. They can also arise from overuse of the joint, such as repetitive motions like throwing a ball, or from twisting the shoulder too forcefully during activities like golf that involve overhead reaching with one arm. These mechanisms of injury highlight the importance of understanding how different activities can strain the shoulder and contribute to potential injuries.

First Aid for Shoulder Injury

The First Aid Treatment for shoulder injuries focuses on minimizing further damage and gradually strengthening the surrounding muscles to prevent re-injury.

> ➢ Limit shoulder use during the initial two days following the injury. After this period, gradually increase shoulder activity, but proceed gently and slowly to avoid re-injury.

➤ Maintain good posture by avoiding slouching. When sitting, support your elbows on chair armrests or a desk to reduce strain on the shoulders.

➤ Apply ice wrapped in a soft cloth for 15 minutes every hour to alleviate pain and swelling. Ice can also be used after exercising or stretching if your shoulder feels sore.

➤ Anti-inflammatory drugs like naproxen sodium and ibuprofen can reduce pain and inflammation associated with shoulder injuries. Acetaminophen can alleviate pain but does not address inflammation.

➤ Lighten backpack loads and avoid prolonged activities that stress the shoulders, such as extended computer use, driving, or heavy weightlifting.

When to See a doctor

You should seek medical attention from a clinician if you experience any of the following symptoms or conditions after sustaining a shoulder injury:

- Shoulder pain accompanied by fever, swelling, or redness.

- Difficulty moving the shoulder or significant limitations in range of motion.

- Persistent shoulder pain lasting more than 2 weeks despite at-home treatment and rest.

- Numbness or tingling sensations radiating down the arm from the shoulder.

Elbow Injuries

Many people have experienced minor elbow injuries, such as bumping their "**funny bone**" at the back of the elbow, which can cause shooting numbness and pain. Although this sensation can be intense, it's generally not serious and will typically resolve on its own.

Other common minor elbow injuries may involve soreness following physical activity. Symptoms of these injuries can include pain, swelling, numbness, tingling, weakness, or decreased range of motion. Fortunately, home treatment methods are often effective in relieving minor elbow aches and pains.

First Aid Procedure for Elbow Injuries

➢ Encourage the injured person to rest the elbow to prevent further strain or damage.

➢ Apply an ice pack or cold compress to the affected area for about 15-20 minutes every few hours during the first 48 hours to reduce pain and swelling. Ensure the ice is wrapped in a cloth to prevent direct skin contact, which can cause ice burns.

➢ Use an elastic bandage to wrap the elbow gently. This can help reduce swelling and provide support.

➢ Keep the injured elbow elevated above heart level, if possible, to further reduce swelling.

➢ Over-the-counter pain relievers such as ibuprofen or acetaminophen can be used to alleviate pain and discomfort. Follow dosage instructions carefully.

➢ Advise the individual to avoid activities that worsen the pain or strain the elbow until it heals.

➢ If the elbow injury is severe, or if there are signs of a fracture (such as deformity, inability to move the elbow, or intense pain), seek immediate medical attention.

➢ Encourage the injured person to follow up with a healthcare professional if symptoms persist or worsen despite home treatment.

Hand Injuries

At some point, most people will encounter hand injuries leading to painful swelling. While routine activities usually don't pose issues, it's not uncommon for symptoms to arise due to everyday wear and tear on our hands.

Hand injuries frequently happen during sports, recreational activities, work tasks, and home-related chores, as well as from accidental falls or physical altercations. According to the Bureau of Labor Statistics, approximately 143,000 hand-related injuries were reported in 2023, resulting in an average loss of five working days per injury in the workplace alone.

First Aid for Hand Injury

When addressing acute hand injuries, follow the PRICE principle, an acronym that stands for protection, rest, ice, and elevation. The aim of PRICE treatment is to alleviate hand pain and swelling, setting the stage for effective rehabilitation if needed.

- ➤ **Protection**: Immediately remove the injured person from the scene to prevent further harm within the first 48 hours post-injury.
- ➤ **Rest**: Advise the individual to refrain from engaging in any activities, including sports, work, or household tasks, following a hand injury.
- ➤ **Ice Application**: To alleviate pain, apply a cold compress or ice for 20 minutes every other hour over a day or two. An effective homemade ice pack can be made by placing crushed ice and water in a plastic bag or cloth, with a damp towel placed between the ice and skin.
- ➤ **Compression**: Apply a pressure or compression bandage to the injured hand to reduce swelling and prevent stiffness. Use a small elastic bandage specifically designed for this type of injury, keeping it on for two to three days post-injury.
- ➤ **Elevation**: Minimize swelling by keeping the injured hand elevated above heart level during the initial hours. Maintain elevation for up to 24 hours whenever possible, ensuring the injured area is also compressed to minimize internal bleeding and swelling

Rib Injuries

A rib fracture, medically known as a broken rib, typically occurs due to car accidents, sports injuries, or other traumatic events. In some cases, a rib can break without direct trauma.

Surgery to repair a rib fracture is uncommon unless the injury has also harmed internal organs. Unlike many other bone fractures, rib fractures usually heal with rest, ice application, and specific breathing exercises. Recovery from a rib fracture generally takes at least a month.

Complications of Broken Ribs

The primary complication of broken ribs is difficulty breathing deeply due to pain. Shallow breathing can cause mucus and moisture buildup in the lungs, increasing the risk of infections like pneumonia. Displaced rib fractures can also harm surrounding tissues or organs, potentially leading to conditions such as collapsed lungs (pneumothorax) or internal bleeding.

Maintaining lung health is crucial during recovery. Practice deep breathing exercises as you heal to prevent respiratory issues. Follow prescribed pain medication to manage discomfort effectively, enabling you to breathe deeply without fear of pain. Taking these measures supports optimal healing and reduces the risk of complications associated with broken ribs.

For initial treatment of a rib injury, follow these steps

➢ Start by applying ice to the injured area. This helps reduce inflammation and pain. Use an ice pack wrapped in a cloth and apply it for about 20-30 minutes.

➢ Over-the-counter pain medication can be given to alleviate pain and discomfort.

➢ If the injury affects the chest and causes pain with movement, wrap an elastic ace bandage around the chest to limit movement and provide support.

➢ Advise the injured person to take shallow breaths and avoid deep breathing to minimize pain.

➢ Loosen the ace bandage around the waist every hour and have the person take a few deep breaths. This can be uncomfortable but is important for lung function.

➢ Apply ice packs wrapped in cloth to the injured area for 20-30 minutes every 2 hours for the first few days to reduce swelling and pain.

➢ Encourage the person to avoid activities that cause pain. Rest and take it slow to allow the injury to heal.

➢ Depending on the severity of the injury, healing may take 4-6 weeks. The pain should gradually decrease over time.

Pelvis Injuries

Managing a casualty with a pelvic injury, especially in remote settings, is critical due to the potential life-threatening nature of these injuries. Understanding the cause, recognition, and appropriate treatment is key.

Anatomy of the Pelvis: The pelvis is a robust, ring-like structure consisting of the ilium bones joined to the sacrum at the base of the spine. The front of this "ring" is completed by the symphysis pubis, a cartilage bridge that allows flexibility for pelvic movement, particularly during childbirth. Interestingly, both males and females have a symphysis pubis, as all fetuses initially develop as females due to carrying the X chromosome.

Concerns with Pelvic Fractures: A fractured pelvis can become unstable, requiring stabilization, especially before moving the casualty. This is crucial because the femoral arteries pass across the front of the pelvis, and movement of fractured bone ends can lead to severe internal bleeding, posing a significant risk.

Understanding these aspects is vital for safely managing pelvic injuries and preventing further complications, particularly in environments where immediate medical assistance may be limited.

The first aid steps for a pelvic injury involve the following:

➤ Approach the injured person carefully, ensuring safety for yourself and the casualty. Assess the situation to determine the severity of the injury and the need for immediate medical assistance.

➤ Encourage the casualty to lie still and avoid unnecessary movement, especially if a pelvic fracture is suspected. If the casualty must be moved, use supportive materials (such as pillows or blankets) to stabilize the pelvis and minimize movement of the injured area.

➤ Apply direct pressure to any external bleeding using a clean cloth or bandage. Avoid applying pressure directly on the pelvis if a fracture is suspected, as this could worsen internal bleeding.

- ➢ Provide reassurance to the casualty to keep them calm. Ensure the injured individual stays warm by wrapping them in a blanket or clothing to avoid shock.
- ➢ Call emergency services or transport the casualty to the nearest medical facility as soon as possible. Inform medical responders about the suspected pelvic injury and any observed symptoms or signs of internal bleeding.
- ➢ Continuously monitor the casualty's condition, looking for signs of shock (such as pale skin, rapid heartbeat, or shallow breathing). Be prepared to provide additional first aid measures based on the casualty's response and medical guidance.

Knee Injuries

The knee joint and its supporting structures are susceptible to injuries caused by various factors such as awkward movements, falls, sudden twists, excessive force, or overuse. These injuries can lead to ligament, tendon, and cartilage tears, as well as patellofemoral pain syndrome.

Seeking prompt medical attention for any knee injury is crucial to improve the chances of a complete recovery. Treatment options may include physiotherapy, arthroscopic surgery, or open surgery, depending on the severity and nature of the injury.

Structure of the Knee

The knee functions as a hinge joint located between the femur (thigh bone) and the tibia and fibula (shin bones). Muscles at the front of the thigh (quadriceps) straighten the leg, while those at the back (hamstrings) allow bending at the knee. The femur's end sits in the shallow cup of the tibia, cushioned by thick cartilage.

The kneecap (patella) rests in a groove at the lower end of the femur. Additional cartilages bolster the joint on each side. Ligaments, tough bands of connective tissue, hold the bones in place. The joint is enclosed within a tough capsule lined with a membrane and filled with lubricating synovial fluid. Bursae, fluid-filled capsules, provide extra cushioning around the joint.

First Aid for Knee Injury

> ➤ If someone sustains a knee injury, it's important to stop any activity immediately. Encourage the person not to try to 'work through' the pain, as this can exacerbate the injury.

> ➤ After stopping the activity, guide the injured person to rest the affected knee. Avoid putting weight on the injured leg to prevent further damage.

> ➤ To reduce pain, swelling, and internal bleeding, apply an ice pack to the injured knee. Use the ice pack for about 15 minutes every couple of hours during the initial 48 to 72 hours post-injury. Ensure the ice pack is wrapped in a cloth or towel to protect the skin from frostbite.

> ➤ Carefully bandage the knee using a firm but not overly tight wrap. Start from above the knee and extend the wrapping down the lower leg to provide support and compression, which helps reduce swelling.

> ➤ Elevate the injured leg to a level above the heart if possible. This positioning can assist in reducing swelling by promoting better circulation and fluid drainage.

> ➤ Do not apply heat to the injured knee during the first 48 to 72 hours. Heat can increase blood flow to the area, which may exacerbate swelling and pain.

> ➤ Encourage the injured person to refrain from consuming alcohol. Alcohol can contribute to increased bleeding and swelling, prolonging the recovery process.

> ➤ Advising against massaging the injured knee is important, as it can further promote bleeding and swelling within the joint. Instead, focus on providing support and following the recommended first aid measures.

Spinal Injuries

Spinal injuries typically result from a significant impact or twisting force, affecting the spinal cord—a complex structure of vertebrae, nerves, and muscles extending from the brainstem to the lower back. The spinal cord serves as a pathway for messages from the brain to other parts of the body. When the spinal cord is severed, blocked, or damaged, areas of the body below the injury site can experience partial or complete paralysis. This loss of communication can profoundly impact motor and sensory functions, leading to varying degrees of impairment depending on the severity and location of the injury. Understanding the implications of spinal injuries is crucial for prompt and appropriate response to minimize potential long-term consequences and provide effective care to those affected.

Symptoms for Spinal Injury

Recognizing symptoms of a spinal injury is crucial in accident scenarios involving the head, neck, or back. If any of these signs are observed, promptly call for an ambulance:

- Weakness or paralysis sensation

- Absence of tactile, thermal, or discomfort perception

- Numbness or tingling, especially in the extremities

- Spasms or uncontrollable motor functions

- Difficulty with balance, walking, or depth perception

- Strong stinging sensation due to nerve damage

- Intense discomfort or compression experienced in the head, neck, or spine

- Clearly twisted neck or back

- Difficulty breathing or clearing throat and lungs

- Loss of bladder or bowel control

If the casualty is responsive

1. Reassure the casualty and advise them not to move, unless they are in immediate danger.

2. Call 911 for emergency help, or ask someone else to make the call.

3. Support the casualty's head, neck, and spine in a straight line to prevent further injury. Kneel or lie behind their head, resting your elbows on the ground or knees to keep your arms steady. Hold each side of their head, ensuring your fingers do not cover their ears.

4. If possible, request assistance from someone to place rolled-up blankets, towels, or clothes on both sides of the head as you ensure the head remains in a neutral position.

5. Continuously monitor the casualty's breathing and level of response until emergency help arrives.

If the casualty is unresponsive

1. Reassure the casualty and avoid moving them unless they are in immediate danger.

2. Call 911 for emergency help, or ask someone else to make the call.

3. Support the casualty's head, neck, and spine in a straight line to prevent further injury. Kneel or lie behind their head, resting your elbows on the ground or knees to stabilize your arms. Hold each side of their head without covering their ears.

4. Use the jaw-thrust technique to open their airway. Place fingertips at the angles of the jaw and gently lift without tilting the neck.

5. Check the casualty's breathing by placing your ear above their mouth for 10 seconds, looking, listening, and feeling for signs of breathing.

6. If the casualty is breathing, continue to support their head and monitor their breathing and response level.

7. If the casualty is unresponsive and not breathing, ensure emergency help has been called and commence CPR immediately. Request assistance in locating and bringing an automated external defibrillator (AED) if available.

CHAPTER 8: COPING WITH MEDICAL EMERGENCIES

Medical emergencies strike unexpectedly, affecting millions of people worldwide each year. These urgent situations can lead to fatalities, often exacerbated by factors such as inadequate healthcare systems, limited access to timely care, and medical errors. In the face of life-threatening conditions, every second counts. Whether it's a heart attack, stroke, severe allergic reaction, or trauma, the immediate response can make the difference between life and death. Patients rely on healthcare professionals, first responders, and bystanders to recognize the signs and take swift action. Internalizing the principles discussed here will enhance your ability to remain composed and proactive in the face of unexpected medical emergencies.

Heart Attacks

A heart attack, also known as **Myocardial Infarction**, occurs when reduced or blocked blood flow to the heart muscle causes damage. This situation is a pressing medical issue that demands prompt care. First aid for a heart attack includes cardiopulmonary resuscitation (CPR), which can significantly increase the chance of saving a person's life.

A heart attack typically manifests as chest pain lasting more than 15 minutes, ranging from mild to severe. However, some individuals may not experience chest pain or pressure. Symptoms can be less apparent in certain groups, particularly women, and may include nausea or brief, sharp pains in the neck, arm, or back.

While some heart attacks occur suddenly, many individuals experience warning signs hours or even days beforehand. This variability underscores the importance of recognizing both typical and atypical symptoms to ensure timely intervention and treatment.

Signs of a heart attack can include

- Chest discomfort marked by feelings of pressure, constriction, squeezing, or throbbing.

- Pain or discomfort that radiates to the shoulder, arm, back, neck, jaw, teeth, or upper abdomen.

- Cold sweats.

- Fatigue.

- Heartburn or indigestion.

- Lightheadedness or sudden dizziness.

- Nausea.

- Shortness of breath.

First Aid for Heart Attack

Here are the first aid steps for someone suspected of having a heart attack, rephrased for clarity and readability:

If you suspect someone is having a heart attack, follow these steps:

➢ Ask the individual to sit, relax, and attempt to remain composed. Loosen any tight clothing to ease discomfort.

➢ Ask if the person takes any chest pain medication, such as nitroglycerin for a known heart condition, and assist them in taking it if available.

➢ If the pain persists after resting or taking nitroglycerin, or if the person is unconscious and unresponsive, call emergency medical services immediately (911 or local emergency number).

➢ If the person is unconscious, not breathing, or has no pulse, start CPR immediately. For infants or children in the same condition, perform 1 minute of CPR before calling emergency services.

➢ If an AED is readily available and the person is unconscious with no pulse, follow the instructions on the AED device.

Strokes

A stroke occurs when blood flow is obstructed to a specific area of the brain, typically due to either a clot or a ruptured blood vessel. This interruption leads to a deprivation of oxygen and nutrients to brain cells, resulting in tissue death and potential brain damage.

There are three primary types of stroke:

1. **Ischemic Stroke**: This type of stroke occurs when a clot blocks blood flow to the brain, cutting off the supply of oxygen and nutrients to brain cells in the affected area.

2. **Hemorrhagic Stroke**: This stroke occurs when a blood vessel bursts or leaks, causing bleeding (hemorrhage) in or around the brain. The sudden pressure from the leaked blood can damage brain cells.

3. **Transient Ischemic Attack** (TIA): Previously known as a mini-stroke, a TIA is caused by temporary blood clots or reduced blood flow to the brain. Unlike a full stroke, TIAs do not typically cause permanent brain damage but are important warning signs of potential stroke risk.

To identify signs of a stroke and take prompt action, remember the acronym **FAST**:

- **Face**: Check for facial changes such as drooping on one side or an uneven smile.

- **Arms**: See if the person can raise both arms and hold them up without drifting.

- **Speech**: Pay attention to speech that sounds slurred or experiences trouble repeating a basic sentence.

- **Time**: If any of these signs are present, call 911 immediately.

After calling 911 for assistance, follow these steps to provide immediate aid:

➢ Keep a composed demeanor to facilitate clear thinking and effective assistance.
➢ Check the surroundings for potential dangers like moving vehicles or hazardous conditions.
➢ Communicate calmly with the individual. Ask their name and assess their responsiveness by requesting them to squeeze your hand.

- If the person is conscious, gently place them on their side with their head and shoulders slightly elevated using a pillow or clothing item for support. Avoid unnecessary movements.
- If clothing is tight or restrictive, such as collars or scarves, loosen them to improve comfort and breathing.
- Cover the person with a blanket or coat if they feel cold to prevent hypothermia.
- Ensure the airway is unobstructed. If there are substances like vomit hindering breathing, place the person on their side (recovery position) to facilitate clearance.
- Comfort the individual by informing them that help is on the way.
- Avoid providing any food or beverages.
- Note any symptoms and observe for changes in the person's condition. Provide detailed information to emergency personnel upon their arrival.
- Record the onset time of symptoms to aid medical responders.

For unconscious individuals:

- Gently position the unconscious person onto their side to maintain an open airway.
- Assess breathing by observing chest movements, listening for breath sounds, and feeling for exhalations against your cheek.
- If there are no signs of breathing, begin CPR (cardiopulmonary resuscitation) as trained or instructed by emergency services.

To place someone in the recovery position when they are unconscious or if their airway is obstructed, follow these steps:

- Kneel beside the person.
- Take the arm farthest from you and position it at a right angle to their body.
- Place their other arm across their chest.
- Keep the leg farthest from you straight, and bend the other knee.
- Support their head and neck, then gently roll the person onto their side. Ensure their bottom leg remains straight while their top leg is bent at the knee, with the knee touching the ground.

- ➢ Tilt their head slightly forward and down to facilitate the drainage of any vomit from the airway.
- ➢ If needed, manually clear the person's mouth to ensure it is free from obstructions.

Asthma

During an asthma attack, the muscles surrounding the air passages in the lungs contract and go into spasm. This spasm causes the airways to narrow, making breathing challenging. Asthma attacks can be triggered by various factors such as a cold, certain medications, cigarette smoke, or allergies. In some cases, asthma attacks occur without any identifiable trigger.

First Aid for Asthma

- ➢ Reassure the person having the asthma attack and encourage them to use their reliever inhaler (typically blue). Guide them to take slow and deep breaths.
- ➢ If they have a spacer available, recommend using it with their inhaler for better effectiveness, especially for young children.
- ➢ If the person does not have an inhaler, immediately call 911 for emergency assistance.
- ➢ Help the person sit comfortably.
- ➢ For a mild attack, it should improve after a few minutes. If not, instruct them to take a puff of their inhaler every 30 to 60 seconds, up to a total of 10 puffs. Assist them if needed.
- ➢ If the attack worsens, they become exhausted, or it's their first attack, call emergency services immediately.
- ➢ Continuously monitor their breathing and responsiveness. If emergency services have not arrived within 15 minutes, repeat step 4.
- ➢ Be prepared to administer CPR if the person becomes unresponsive.
- ➢ If symptoms improve and emergency services are not required, advise the person to seek urgent same-day medical attention from their GP or asthma nurse.

Allergic Reactions

Your body's immune system produces antibodies to combat foreign substances and prevent illness. However, sometimes the immune system mistakenly identifies harmless substances as threats, triggering what we call an allergic reaction. These substances, known as allergens, can range from food and medications to environmental factors.

Exposure to allergens can result in mild symptoms such as skin irritation, watery eyes, or sneezing. For some individuals, allergies can escalate to a severe condition called anaphylaxis. Anaphylaxis is life-threatening and involves shock, a sudden drop in blood pressure, and breathing difficulties, which can progress to respiratory failure and cardiac arrest.

If you or someone else is experiencing anaphylaxis, it's essential to immediately call 911 or your local emergency services for prompt medical intervention. Early treatment is critical in managing this severe allergic reaction and preventing serious complications.

The most severe allergic reactions can trigger anaphylaxis, a rapid and potentially life-threatening response that can lead to loss of consciousness, respiratory distress, and cardiac arrest if left untreated.

Recognizable signs of anaphylaxis include:

- Skin reactions such as hives, itching, or pale skin

- Wheezing or difficulty breathing

- Feeling lightheaded, dizzy, or faint

- Swelling of the face

- Nausea

- Weak and rapid pulse

First Aid

If you're with someone experiencing an allergic reaction with signs of anaphylaxis, follow these steps:

> ➢ Promptly dial 911 or the emergency number for medical assistance in your area.

- ➤ Check if the person has an epinephrine autoinjector (EpiPen, Auvi-Q, others) for treating allergic reactions.
- ➤ If needed, assist the person in using the autoinjector. Typically, this involves pressing the autoinjector against the person's thigh.
- ➤ Have the person lie face up and remain still.
- ➤ Loosen any tight attire and wrap the individual in a blanket. Avoid giving them anything to drink.
- ➤ If there's vomiting or bleeding from the mouth, turn the person to their side to prevent choking.
- ➤ If the person is not breathing, coughing, or moving, begin CPR with uninterrupted chest compressions at a rate of about 100 per minute until paramedics arrive.
- ➤ Seek emergency treatment even if symptoms improve. Anaphylaxis symptoms can recur, and monitoring in a hospital for several hours is typically necessary.

Meningitis

Meningitis is characterized by inflammation of the protective membranes surrounding the brain and spinal cord, known as the meninges. This inflammation typically results from an infection, though the specific cause can vary. While the meningitis vaccine is now part of routine immunizations, it does not offer protection against all strains of the disease.

Meningococcal Group B is the most prevalent cause of meningitis, and a vaccine targeting this strain is readily available. Meningitis is commonly categorized as either bacterial or viral, although it can be caused by various microbes. Viral meningitis, while unpleasant, is seldom life-threatening and often leads to full recovery. In contrast, bacterial meningitis is more severe and can have lasting or fatal consequences.

Signs and Symptoms of Meningitis

When assessing for meningitis, watch out for the following signs and symptoms:

- • Feeling very unwell, resembling a flu-like illness, often accompanied by a high temperature

- Skin that appears mottled or very pale

- Cold hands and feet

- Joint and limb pain

- As the infection progresses, individuals may experience a severe headache

- Stiffness in the neck

- Vomiting

- Sensitivity to light (photophobia)

- Drowsiness

- In babies, be alert for a shrill, moaning, or whining cry, coupled with limpness and a firm or protruding area on the crown of the head (fontanelle).

- Later on, a distinctive rash of red or purple spots that do not fade when pressed

First aid for suspected meningitis involves the following steps:

- Be alert for signs of meningitis, which can include severe headache, stiff neck, fever, confusion, sensitivity to light, nausea, and rash.

- Immediately call emergency services (911 or local equivalent) if you suspect someone has meningitis. Time is critical for effective treatment.

- Ensure the individual remains composed and at ease until medical aid arrives. Recommend resting in a serene environment with subdued lighting.

- Check the person's vital signs regularly. Be prepared to provide CPR if they become unresponsive and stop breathing.

- Avoid giving the person anything to eat or drink until medical professionals arrive and assess the situation.

- If you must come into contact with the person's bodily fluids (e.g., saliva, mucus), wear gloves and wash your hands thoroughly afterward.

- Once medical help arrives, provide them with all relevant information and follow their instructions closely.

Diabetic Emergencies

Diabetes is a chronic condition where the body struggles to process glucose (sugar) in the bloodstream. The pancreas, an organ in the body, normally produces insulin, a hormone responsible for moving glucose from the bloodstream into cells for energy use. In diabetes, either the pancreas doesn't produce enough insulin, or the body's cells don't respond effectively to insulin. This leads to elevated levels of glucose in the bloodstream.

Types of Diabetes

Diabetes is categorized into two main types based on how the body handles blood sugar:

Hyperglycemia: Hyperglycemia occurs when there are lower levels of insulin in the body, leading to higher blood sugar levels. This can happen due to various reasons such as excessive food intake, insufficient medication, decreased physical activity, or experiencing physical or emotional stress. Hyperglycemia develops gradually and is not typically considered a first aid emergency.

When hyperglycemia occurs, the body's cells are unable to access the sugar they need for energy, even though there is excess sugar in the bloodstream. To compensate, the body breaks down other sources of energy, resulting in the buildup of waste products and illness. A distinct fruity or sweet odor in the breath may be present, indicating a potential diabetic emergency known as diabetic coma.

Hypoglycemia: Hypoglycemia occurs when insulin levels are too high relative to blood sugar levels, causing a rapid depletion of sugar in the blood. This can happen if a person misses a meal or snack, engages in excessive exercise, vomits, or takes an excess amount of medication. In hypoglycemia, the brain does not receive enough sugar to function properly, resulting in a critical condition known as insulin shock. Hypoglycemia develops quickly and is the primary cause of diabetic emergencies.

First Aid Treatment for Diabetes

High Blood Sugar (Hyperglycemia):

➢ If the patient has diabetes medication and requires assistance, ask them if they need help administering it. Only assist if the patient requests it to ensure they maintain control over their treatment regimen.

➢ Advise the patient to drink water to help dilute excess sugar in the bloodstream and support kidney function in removing glucose through urine.

➢ If the patient's symptoms of hyperglycemia worsen (such as excessive thirst, frequent urination, fatigue, or confusion), advise them to seek immediate medical attention to prevent complications like diabetic ketoacidosis.

➢ For individuals not diagnosed with diabetes but experiencing symptoms of high blood sugar, recommend they seek medical evaluation to determine the underlying cause and receive appropriate treatment.

Low Blood Sugar (Hypoglycemia):

➢ Assist the patient in sitting or lying down comfortably to prevent falls and injuries due to dizziness or weakness caused by low blood sugar.

➢ Offer verbal reassurance to help calm the patient, as hypoglycemia can cause anxiety, confusion, and irritability.

➢ Check and loosen any tight clothing to ensure unrestricted blood flow and comfort for the patient.

➢ Offer fast-acting sources of sugar to raise blood glucose levels quickly. This can include fruit juice, regular soft drinks (avoid diet versions), sugar, jellybeans, or glucose tablets.

➢ Continue providing sugar every 15 minutes until the patient's symptoms improve. Monitor the patient's response and adjust sugar intake accordingly.

➢ Once the patient's blood sugar stabilizes, offer carbohydrates for sustained energy. This can include a balanced meal like a sandwich, milk, fresh or dried fruit, or crackers with cheese.

➢ If the patient's condition does not improve or if they lose consciousness due to severe hypoglycemia, call emergency services (911) immediately for professional medical intervention and treatment.

Poisoning

Poisoning can result from swallowing, inhaling, touching, or injecting various substances like drugs, chemicals, venoms, or gases, leading to injury or death. Some substances are only toxic in higher concentrations, while others pose a threat primarily through ingestion. Children are especially vulnerable to even small amounts of certain substances.

Treatment for suspected poisoning depends on several factors:

- The person's symptoms.

- Their age.

- Knowledge of the type and amount of the substance involved.

If you suspect poisoning, contact Poison Help at 800-222-1222 in the United States or your regional poison control center immediately. Consider displaying the poison control number prominently in your home using a magnet or sticker. Poison control centers offer valuable information and may advise that home observation is sufficient in many cases.

When to seek emergency help

Know when to seek emergency help by calling 911 or your local emergency number immediately if the person:

- Is drowsy or unconscious.

- Is having difficulty breathing or has stopped breathing.

- Appears uncontrollably restless or agitated.

- Is experiencing seizures.

- Has intentionally or accidentally overdosed on medications or substances (often involving larger amounts, possibly with alcohol).

For situations where the person is stable with no symptoms and is being transported to the local emergency department, consider calling Poison Help at 800-222-1222 in the United States or your regional poison control center. Be prepared to provide detailed information about the person's symptoms, age, weight, current medications, and any known information about the poison. If possible, have the pill bottle, medicine package, or suspected container nearby to reference its label when speaking with the poison control center.

Signs and Symptoms of Poisoning

Poisoning can present symptoms that resemble other conditions like seizures, alcohol intoxication, stroke, or insulin reactions. Common symptoms of poisoning include:

- Redness or burns surrounding the mouth and lips.

- Breath that smells of chemicals, such as gasoline or paint thinner.

- Vomiting.

- Difficulty breathing.

- Drowsiness.

- Confusion or altered mental status.

If you suspect poisoning, remain vigilant for clues such as empty pill bottles or packages, scattered pills, and evidence of burns, stains, or odors on the person or nearby objects. When dealing with a child, consider the possibility of accidental ingestion of medicated patches, prescription medicines, or even swallowing a button battery. Early recognition and prompt action are crucial when poisoning is suspected.

First Aid for Treatment

1. **Swallowed Poison**: Remove any remaining substance from the person's mouth. For household cleaners or chemicals, refer to the label for accidental poisoning instructions.

2. **Poison on the Skin**: Use gloves to remove contaminated clothing and rinse the affected skin with water for 15 to 20 minutes in a shower or with a hose.

3. **Poison in the Eye**: Gently flush the eye with cool or lukewarm water continuously for 20 minutes or until help arrives.

4. **Button Batteries**: If a child swallows a button battery, seek immediate emergency X-ray to locate it. Remove promptly if stuck in the esophagus; if in the stomach, it usually passes through.

5. **Medicated Patches**: Check the child's skin for medicated patches and remove any found. Inspect the roof of the mouth for patches that may have become lodged.

6. **Inhaled Poison**: Move the person to fresh air quickly and turn the head to the side if vomiting occurs to prevent choking.

7. **Cardiopulmonary Resuscitation (CPR)**: Start CPR immediately if the person shows no signs of life (movement, breathing, coughing).

8. **Seek Professional Help**: Call Poison Help at 800-222-1222 (in the U.S.) or your local poison control center for further instructions. Gather pill bottles, packages, or containers with labels and any relevant information to provide to the ambulance team.

Emergency Childbirth

Childbirth is typically a gradual process that unfolds over several hours, allowing time to seek the assistance of a midwife or transport the woman to a birthing facility. However, in some instances, childbirth can occur suddenly and unexpectedly, known as an "emergency birth," often taking place in a location that was not originally planned for.

During childbirth, the body naturally progresses through three phases. The first phase involves contractions and the breaking of the woman's water. In the second phase, the woman actively pushes to deliver the baby. The final stage occurs when the woman delivers the afterbirth, which includes the placenta.

In cases of emergency birth, the role of the first aid provider is to offer supportive care to the woman throughout the process. This may involve assisting with the delivery and ensuring the safety and well-being of both the mother and the newborn.

Guidelines

- Support the woman in contacting her chosen birthing partner, as their continuous support during labour contributes to a positive childbirth experience.

- Encourage an upright position (sitting, standing, or walking) during the first stage of labour, as it may help shorten its duration.

- Provide lower back massage during labour to reduce pain intensity.

- Promote relaxation techniques such as yoga, music, or general relaxation to reduce pain and improve the birthing experience.

- Encourage skin-to-skin contact between the mother and baby to improve breastfeeding and enhance infant and maternal outcomes.

Good Practice Points

- Ensure the dignity and safety of the woman by managing the scene appropriately and providing emotional support and comfort.

- Support the woman in finding positions that are most comfortable, even if her waters have broken (amniotic sac is broken).

- Allow the woman to drink or eat if desired during labour.

- Maintain hygiene by using gloves and clean cloths or towels under the mother and for wrapping the newborn.

- After delivery, assess the responsiveness, breathing, and bleeding of both the woman and the baby.

- If the baby is responsive and breathing normally, keep the baby warm and dry without immediately cutting the umbilical cord.

- If the baby is unresponsive, rub the baby dry and stimulate breathing by tapping the soles of its feet. Initiate CPR promptly if necessary. If the umbilical cord impedes resuscitation efforts, it may need to be cut.

- If cutting the umbilical cord is required, tie it twice with a ribbon, spaced a hand-width apart, and cut between the ribbons, with the first ribbon about a hand-width from the baby's belly.

- These guidelines and practices aim to ensure a supportive and safe environment during childbirth, prioritizing the well-being of both the mother and baby.

First Aid

➢ When attending to a woman in labor, prioritize her needs as well as those of the baby being born.

➢ Coordinate with medical facilities, EMS, or a midwife based on the woman's preferences and follow their guidance. Assist the woman in contacting her chosen birthing partner for additional support.

➢ Create a calm and private environment for the woman during the initial phase of childbirth. Help her find a comfortable position, which could be sitting, standing, or moving around. Offer methods like massage or relaxation techniques to reduce pain and anxiety.

➢ In the active phase of labor, assist the woman in assuming a comfortable position, preferably upright. If lying on her back, place a small pillow under her right hip to avoid compressing important blood vessels.

➢ Prepare for delivery by washing hands thoroughly and placing a clean cloth under the woman where the baby will be born. Provide support as the woman prepares to push during delivery.

➢ Monitor the baby's head as it emerges to ensure gentle and careful handling due to its slippery nature.

➢ Immediately after birth, use a clean cloth to dry and wrap the baby, covering its head to maintain warmth. Place the baby on the mother's chest or abdomen as soon as possible for skin-to-skin contact.

➢ During the final phase of childbirth, support the woman as she delivers the afterbirth (placenta). Keep the afterbirth intact for examination by healthcare professionals.

➢ Monitor the woman for signs of excessive bleeding after delivery. While mild bleeding is normal, severe bleeding requires immediate attention. Help the woman lie down, keep warm, and seek medical help promptly if needed.

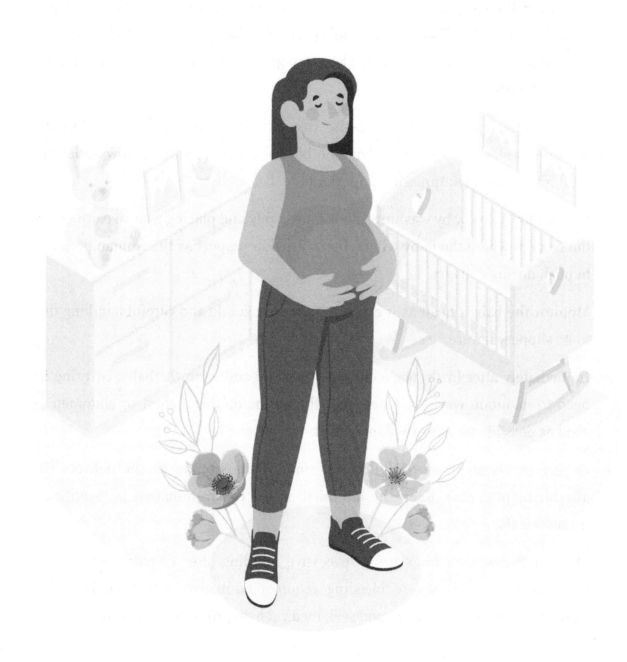

CHAPTER 9: PEDIATRIC FIRST AID

Pediatric first aid training equips individuals with essential skills tailored for treating children under the age of 16. This specialized form of first aid is crucial in environments where children are present, such as homes, schools, daycare centers, and recreational facilities. The techniques learned in pediatric first aid address the unique needs and vulnerabilities of children, ensuring timely and effective response to emergencies and injuries specific to this age group. In this chapter, we explore the fundamentals of pediatric first aid, focusing on key skills and strategies for managing common childhood injuries and medical emergencies.

Caring for Unwell Children and Babies

It's common for children to experience illness periodically, and parents often feel concerned when their usually happy child appears sad and lacking in energy. Fortunately, most infections are temporary and pass relatively quickly. In fact, going through these illnesses can actually strengthen a child's immune system, making them more resilient to similar infections in the future.

If your child isn't feeling well, it's important to take the following steps:

1. When in doubt about your child's health, always consult with a healthcare professional for advice and reassurance.

2. Many childhood illnesses resolve on their own and can be managed at home. However, be cautious with medications like paracetamol and ibuprofen, as they may not be suitable for all children. Seek guidance from a pharmacist.

3. Antibiotics are effective only against bacterial infections, not viral illnesses which are common in childhood.

4. Trust your instincts if you suspect a serious illness and seek prompt medical help.

5. Learn basic first aid skills to manage minor injuries like cuts and scrapes.

6. Be prepared for emergencies by knowing what to do and staying calm to provide the best care for your child.

Recognizing when your child is unwell can sometimes be challenging, as their condition may fluctuate rapidly. Here are some considerations if you suspect your child is ill:

- Watch for physical signs like vomiting, high temperature, coughing, or changes in behavior such as crying, irritability, refusal of food and drink, or appearing lethargic and drowsy.

- Trust your instincts as a parent; you know your child best and can identify unusual or concerning behaviors.

- If uncertain about your child's health or if symptoms persist, contact your GP or health visitor. If unable to reach them, contact your local accident and emergency department.

Certain symptoms should always be taken seriously:

- Your baby appears floppy when picked up.

- Your baby refuses to drink for more than eight hours, with food intake becoming less important.

- A bulging fontanelle (soft spot on a baby's head), weak high-pitched continuous crying, or repeated vomiting, especially of green bile.

- High temperatures above 38 degrees for infants under three months or above 39 degrees for infants aged three to six months.

- Signs of circulation issues like a high temperature coupled with cold feet or hands, or the appearance of a fit or seizure.

- Noticeable changes in skin color (blue, mottled, or very pale) or difficulty breathing, including rapid or labored breathing, grunting, or signs of respiratory distress.

- Signs of a stiff neck, unusual drowsiness or difficulty waking, or confusion.

- A child's inability to stay awake after being roused, or the appearance of a spotty purple rash, which could indicate meningitis and warrants urgent medical attention.

First Aid Care

Caring for a sick child can be challenging, but there are ways to help them feel better and recover:

- Listen to your child's needs and preferences. If they don't want to stay in bed, consider letting them rest on a sofa or armchair closer to you for companionship.
- Ensure the room is comfortably ventilated. Avoid making it too warm or drafty, as this can exacerbate their discomfort.
- Offer plenty of fluids to keep them hydrated. Don't worry about food initially; focus on fluids unless they express an appetite.
- Keep them entertained with quiet games and stories to provide comfort and distraction.
- Encourage rest and napping as needed. Reading a calming story can aid in relaxation.
- Avoid sleeping on a sofa with a sick child, as this poses risks, especially when both of you are tired.

Pediatric CPR

Before performing CPR on a child or baby, follow these steps:

1. Check the area for safety and form an initial impression of the situation. Obtain consent from the parent or guardian if present and use personal protective equipment (PPE) if available.

2. Check for Responsiveness:

   - For a child: Shout to get their attention using their name if known. If there is no response, gently tap their shoulder and shout again while checking for breathing or signs of life-threatening conditions.

   - For a baby: Shout to get their attention using their name if known. If there is no response, gently tap the bottom of their foot and shout again while checking for breathing or signs of life-threatening conditions.

   - Assess responsiveness for a maximum of 10 seconds.

3. If the child or baby is unresponsive and not breathing or only gasping, immediately call 9-1-1 and retrieve any necessary equipment, or instruct someone else to do so.

Performing CPR on a child or baby involves specific steps:

Positioning: Place the child or baby on their back on a firm, flat surface. Kneel beside the child or stand/kneel to the side of the baby with hips at a slight angle.

Chest Compressions: For a child, use two hands in the center of the chest, keeping arms straight and shoulders over hands. Compress the chest about 2 inches deep at a rate of 100 to 120 compressions per minute. For a small child, use one hand in the center of the chest and compress similarly. Use two thumbs on the center of the chest just below the nipple line, or use two fingers parallel to the chest. Compress about 1 ½ inches deep at a rate of 100 to 120 compressions per minute.

Giving Breaths: Open the airway: tilt the head back slightly for a child and to a neutral position for a baby. Deliver breaths into the mouth/nose for about 1 second, ensuring chest rise with each breath.

Continued Cycle:

Alternate between 30 chest compressions and 2 breaths continuously until:

- Signs of life are evident.
- An AED (Automated External Defibrillator) is available.
- Another trained responder takes over.
- EMS personnel arrive and assume responsibility for providing care.
- You are alone and too fatigued to continue.
- The scene becomes unsafe.

Approximately 2 minutes of CPR have been performed, and you need to call 911 while caring for a baby.

Choking Procedures

Knowing what to do if your baby is choking is crucial for caregivers. Acting swiftly can potentially dislodge an obstructed airway and save precious seconds. Below are important steps to assist a baby (under 12 months old) who is choking, along with what actions to avoid and tips to prevent choking accidents at home.

First Aid steps

- ➤ **Step 1**: Verify Choking Ensure your baby is actually choking. If your baby is coughing or gagging but able to make noise and breathe, they are likely not choking. True choking is indicated by an inability to cry, cough, or make noise due to a completely obstructed airway.

- ➤ **Step 2**: Call 911 Have someone call 911 or local emergency services while you attend to your baby. Provide updates to the operator and notify them if your baby becomes unconscious during the process.

- ➤ **Step 3**: Perform Back Blows Place your baby face down on your forearm with their head lower than their body. Support them on your thigh and deliver five quick and strong blows between the shoulder blades using the heel of your hand. This action aims to dislodge the obstructing object.

- ➤ **Step 4**: Perform Chest Thrusts Turn your baby over onto their back with their head lower than their chest. Use your index and middle fingers to locate the breastbone (between and slightly below the nipples) and press down five times with enough force to depress the chest about one-third. This helps push air from the lungs into the airway to expel the object.

- ➤ **Step 5**: Repeat if Necessary If the object remains lodged, repeat back blows followed by chest thrusts. Notify the 911 operator immediately if your baby loses consciousness during these steps.

Dehydration

Dehydration in children typically occurs due to vomiting, diarrhea, or a combination of both. It can also happen when children refuse to drink because of mouth sores or a sore throat. Additionally, dehydration may result from exposure to hot weather or excessive physical activity.

How to Treat Dehydration

Treating dehydration depends on its severity. Mild dehydration can typically be managed at home by providing extra fluids. Children with more severe dehydration may require treatment in the emergency room or hospital.

For mild dehydration, oral rehydration is recommended. This involves giving oral rehydration solution like Pedialyte, Enfalyte, or a similar store brand. These solutions contain the right balance of water, sugar, and salt to address dehydration. They are available over-the-counter at drugstores or supermarkets. If oral rehydration solution is not accessible, consult your doctor for alternative options or other liquids that can help manage dehydration.

If your child has mild dehydration and you've been advised by your doctor to treat them at home, follow these guidelines:

> ➢ Offer your child small, frequent sips of oral rehydration solution. For babies, this can be 1–2 teaspoons (5–10 milliliters) every few minutes, while older kids can have 1–2 tablespoons (15–30 milliliters) at a time.

> ➢ Breastfed babies or those on formula can continue their usual feeding, provided they are not repeatedly vomiting.

> ➢ Older children can have electrolyte ice pops to help with hydration.

> ➢ Encourage your child to eat their regular diet unless advised otherwise by the doctor. Initially, they may not have much of an appetite, but as long as they are drinking, it's acceptable if solid foods are consumed in smaller amounts.

> ➢ As your child's condition improves and their appetite returns, gradually decrease the amount of oral rehydration solution and increase their intake of regular food and drink.

> ➢ Avoid giving babies plain water instead of oral rehydration solution, as it lacks the necessary nutrients for treating dehydration in infants.

> ➢ Refrain from offering sports drinks, soda, or undiluted juice, as they contain excessive sugar that can exacerbate symptoms.

➤ Do not administer medications for diarrhea or vomiting without the doctor's recommendation.

Here are signs that indicate you should call your doctor for your child:

- If your child refuses to drink anything for more than a few hours.

- If your child is under 1 year old and has been drinking only oral rehydration solution (no breast milk or formula) for 24 hours.

- If your child vomits frequently, more than a few times within 24 hours, especially if the vomit is bright green, red, or brown in color.

- If your child hasn't started eating any food within 3–4 days.

- If your child shows signs of dehydration such as a dry mouth, decreased urination (or fewer wet diapers in babies), fewer tears, or a sunken soft spot (in babies).

- If your child is unusually cranky, fussy, or less active.

- If your child's situation shows no signs of getting better.

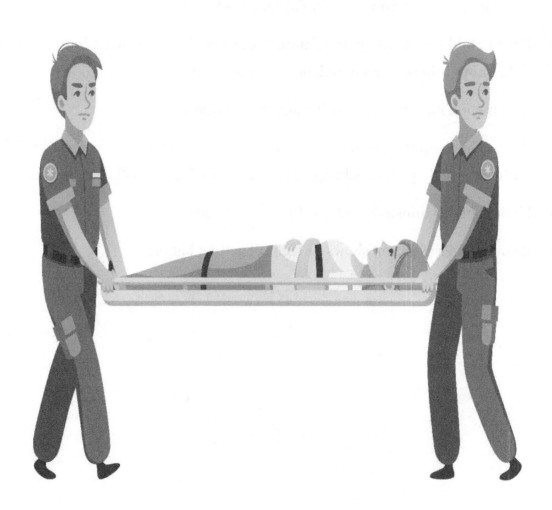

CHAPTER 10: ENVIRONMENTAL HAZARDS

 In today's world, understanding and preparing for environmental emergencies are essential skills for everyone. Many of these emergencies can be prevented by recognizing potential dangers and planning for the possibility of delayed medical assistance. To effectively prepare for such situations, individuals must become acquainted with their surroundings and anticipate the challenges they may encounter. This chapter explores various environmental hazards and provides practical guidance on how to identify and mitigate risks.

Lightning Safety

Lightning occurs when positively charged particles form within a cloud and interact with negatively charged particles, resulting in a powerful discharge known as a lightning strike. This discharge can also occur between charged clouds or between a cloud and the earth's surface. Lightning seeks to discharge or "ground" itself, often targeting prominent objects like lightning rods on buildings, solitary trees, or even people due to their height and conductivity.

First Aid for Lightning

First aid for a casualty struck by lightning involves several important steps:

➤ Dial 911 immediately to summon emergency assistance. Provide clear directions to your location and details about the injured person. Using a mobile phone or cordless telephone during a storm poses no significant safety risk.

➤ Prioritize safety for both the victim and yourself. Be cautious of ongoing lightning danger, especially if you're in a high-risk area like an open field or near isolated trees. Consider moving to a safer location if necessary, but avoid moving victims who are bleeding or may have broken bones.

➤ Check for signs of life. Look for breathing and a pulse—check the carotid artery in the neck or femoral artery in the groin for a pulse. If the person is breathing normally, assess for other injuries such as burns or shock. Provide basic first aid for these injuries and protect against hypothermia if the environment is cold and wet.

- Wear gloves from your first aid kit to protect against cross-contamination, especially if the casualty has multiple burns or injuries.

- Verify that the casualty's airway is clear and confirm if they are breathing.

- If the casualty is not breathing, call emergency services 911 and begin CPR immediately. Lightning strikes can cause prolonged CPR needs due to potential brain damage affecting breathing regulation.

- Assess for spinal injuries if the casualty was thrown by the lightning strike. Note any abnormalities and communicate these to paramedics upon their arrival.

- Expose burns to running water for at least 20 minutes and cover with a sterile dressing to prevent infection. Check the entire body for burns, especially around jewelry, buckles, fingers, and toes.

- Lightning strikes can damage delicate parts like the eyes and ears, potentially causing temporary or permanent blindness or deafness. Communicate sensitively with the casualty.

- Be aware that casualties may experience confusion, nausea, or temporary memory loss. Provide reassurance and keep them calm.

- Stay with the casualty, offering reassurance and monitoring their condition until medical help arrives.

- If there are multiple casualties, prioritize treatment based on urgency. Attend first to casualties who are not breathing.

- Be prepared to address shock in any casualty. Keep conscious casualties on their back with elevated feet and unconscious casualties in the recovery position while awaiting medical assistance.

Drowning

In hot weather or during a heatwave, many people seek relief by swimming in open water. However, it's crucial to be aware of the dangers associated with open water swimming and to understand first aid for drowning incidents. Drowning occurs when someone struggles to breathe because their nose and mouth are submerged in a liquid. Unlike what is often portrayed on TV, drowning may not involve loud calls for help and can go unnoticed even if friends or family are nearby.

To avoid dangers near open water, follow these important guidelines:

1. When swimming outdoors, be cautious of cold water and strong currents, which can pose risks even for proficient swimmers. Always adhere to signs indicating unsafe swimming areas.

2. Water is significantly colder than the air, even on warm days, and can lead to hypothermia after leaving the water. Dry off thoroughly and avoid swimming if the water feels too cold.

3. Stick to shallow areas and remain within your depth. Stay near the shore or edge of the water to ensure a safe return if needed.

4. Keep a close watch on children and young individuals near water at all times. Only swim or paddle in designated areas with lifeguards nearby. When open water swimming, always have a companion with you for safety in case of emergencies.

When rescuing a casualty, ensure your own safety first.

➤ After bringing the casualty out of the water, conduct a primary survey. If the casualty is unresponsive and not breathing, instruct a helper to call emergency services (911) while you initiate CPR. If available, have the helper locate and bring a defibrillator.

➤ If alone, use a hands-free speakerphone to communicate with emergency services while performing CPR.

➤ Begin with checking and clearing the airway before delivering five initial rescue breaths. Position the head with one hand on the forehead and two fingers under the chin, then provide rescue breaths.

➤ Next, start chest compressions by kneeling beside the casualty and placing the heel of one hand in the center of the chest, interlocking fingers and keeping arms straight. Perform compressions at a rate of 100-120 per minute, following the beat of "Staying Alive."

➤ Continue CPR until emergency help arrives, signs of life return, you are too exhausted to continue (if a helper is available, switch every one-to-two minutes), or a defibrillator becomes available.

➤ Be prepared for the casualty to expel stomach contents and roll them onto their side to clear the airway.

➤ If the casualty shows signs of responsiveness, place them in the recovery position and monitor their condition. Treat for hypothermia by covering with warm clothes and blankets.

➤ Seek medical advice for individuals who have experienced near-drowning, even if they appear well initially.

➤ If a defibrillator is used, leave it attached until medical professionals take over.

Here are six important points to understand about drowning:

- Despite being surrounded by water, most drownings actually occur inland, in places like quarries, canals, lakes, and reservoirs where there are no lifeguards or immediate assistance available. It's crucial not to enter the water unless it's a designated swimming area, even on hot days.

- Approximately half of the individuals who drowned had not planned to go into the water. Many drownings happen during everyday activities like walking near water bodies, where individuals may accidentally fall in or attempt risky rescues. It's important to assess the dangers before taking action in emergencies involving water.

- Men, especially younger men aged 20-29, are at a significantly higher risk of drowning compared to women. This demographic is four times more likely to drown, emphasizing the importance of water safety awareness among this group.

- Alcohol contributes to a substantial portion of drownings, with about one in three cases involving alcohol consumption. Drinking can impair judgment and increase risk-taking behaviors, making swimming especially dangerous when intoxicated.

- Drowning does not resemble dramatic scenes from movies. It often occurs silently and quickly, without the typical signs of distress like splashing or screaming. Vigilance is essential to recognize the subtle signs of drowning, such as struggling to breathe and staying at or below the water's surface.

- A drowning person will typically bob below the water's surface and resurface briefly in an attempt to breathe. They may appear to be struggling just to inhale and exhale, without the energy to call for help or make significant movements.

Poisonous Plants

Poisonous plants have historically been a common hazard in daily life. In the nineteenth century, incidents of plant poisonings rose dramatically as people relied on natural vegetation for food sources. Today, the presence of potentially dangerous plants remains prevalent. They are often integrated into indoor interiorscapes and outdoor landscaping. This issue has been exacerbated by the introduction of numerous exotic plant species from around the globe into cultivated environments. Recent research indicates that approximately 3.5% of all poisonings in the United States can be attributed to plant exposure.

Poison Ivy, Poison Oak, and Poison Sumac: These plants contain urushiol, an oily sap that triggers allergic reactions like red, swollen, and itchy skin. Poison Ivy grows over most of the U.S., with vine-like growth in some regions and shrub-like in others. Poison Oak resembles oak leaves and is more common in the West. Poison Sumac is found in wet areas nationwide and requires medical attention for severe rashes.

Giant Hogweed: This plant is tall with umbrella-shaped white flowers, deep creased leaves, and hairy stems. Its sap can cause severe skin reactions and damage vision upon sunlight exposure.

Stinging Nettle: Identified by unbranched patches of stems up to 4-6 feet tall, its tiny hairs contain formic acid causing painful skin reactions on contact.

Australian Stinging Tree: Contains neurotoxins causing prolonged pain upon contact, injecting poison similar to that found in spiders and cone snails.

Wild Parsnip: Recognizable by yellow umbrella-like flowers, its sap causes a skin rash upon sunlight exposure. Common in fields, roadsides, and Midwestern prairies.

Poison Hemlock: Resembling wild carrot with distinctive purple-spotted stems and ridged fruits, it can poison humans and livestock through ingestion or skin contact with its oils.

Foxglove: Known for bell-shaped flowers in various colors, its entire structure is poisonous and can affect heart function.

Bitter Nightshade: A woody perennial with purple flowers and red berries containing solanine, ingestion of which can cause various symptoms requiring immediate medical attention.

First Aid for Poisonous Plants

First aid for workers who have encountered poisonous plants involves several important steps:

- Immediately rinse the affected skin with rubbing alcohol, poison plant washes, degreasing soap (like dishwashing soap), or detergent along with lots of water.
- Rinse frequently to prevent wash solutions from drying on the skin and spreading the urushiol, an oil in the plant that causes contact dermatitis.
- Scrub under nails using a brush to remove any traces of the plant oil.
- Apply wet compresses, calamine lotion, or hydrocortisone cream to the affected skin to alleviate itching and blistering.
- Follow the instructions on creams and lotions carefully and avoid applying them to broken skin like open blisters.
- Consider taking oatmeal baths to relieve itching.
- Take an antihistamine such as diphenhydramine (e.g., Benadryl) as directed to help reduce itching, but be cautious as antihistamines may cause drowsiness.
- If children come into contact with contaminated work clothing, consult a pediatrician for appropriate dosage of antihistamine.
- Seek medical assistance in severe cases or if the rash appears on the face or genitals.
- Call 911 or go to a hospital emergency room immediately if experiencing severe allergic reactions like swelling or difficulty breathing, especially if there's a history of severe reactions to poisonous plants in the past.

CHAPTER 11: DEALING WITH BITES AND STINGS

Most insect bites and stings are mild and can be managed effectively at home. These encounters often result in temporary symptoms like itching, swelling, and stinging, which typically resolve within a day or two. However, in certain cases, bites and stings can cause discomfort or allergic reactions that require specific attention and care. This chapter explores practical strategies for identifying, treating, and preventing common bites and stings encountered in everyday situations.

Animal Bites

The majority of animal bites are inflicted by pets, with dog bites being particularly common and often affecting children. Children are more likely than adults to be bitten on the face, head, or neck by dogs. Cat bites, although less frequent, carry a higher risk of infection due to the longer and sharper teeth that can cause deeper puncture wounds. Other animal bites typically come from stray or wild animals like skunks, raccoons, foxes, and bats. Puncture wounds caused by bites are more prone to infection. Some animals may carry the rabies virus, which, although rare, can be deadly if transmitted to humans.

First Aid for Animal Bites

First aid for minor bite wounds involves taking immediate steps to prevent infection and promote healing, especially when the skin is slightly broken or the bite is from a vaccinated domestic animal or human, like a child. Here's what you can do:

➢ Use soapy water to clean the bite wound thoroughly. This aids in eliminating bacteria, thereby lowering the chances of infection.

➢ After cleaning, apply an antibiotic cream like bacitracin to the affected area. This aids in warding off infections and stimulates the healing process.

➢ Once the wound is cleaned and treated with antibiotic cream, cover it with a clean bandage to protect against further contamination.

➤ Monitor the bite wound for signs of infection, such as increased redness, warmth, pain, pus, or bleeding. If you notice these symptoms, it's important to promptly seek medical help.

➤ If the bite is on the hand or finger, contact your doctor for further evaluation and possible antibiotic treatment, as infections in these areas can be more serious.

In cases of severe bite wounds, which involve deep tearing or significant bleeding, immediate medical attention is crucial:

➤ Apply firm pressure with a clean, dry cloth to the affected area to control bleeding until medical help arrives.

➤ Due to the severity of severe bite wounds, it's essential to seek prompt medical attention for proper evaluation and treatment.

Insect Stings

In the United States, encountering animal and insect bites or stings is common. Some of these incidents can be managed on the spot using supplies from a first aid kit. For certain bites and stings, acting swiftly is crucial. This may involve applying pressure bandages and keeping the affected person still until medical assistance is available. It's important to remain calm and reassure the individual. Avoid using tourniquets or attempting to cut the wound.

Seek immediate medical attention by calling 911 for an ambulance in case of an emergency. If the person collapses or stops breathing, CPR (cardiopulmonary resuscitation) may be necessary until help arrives.

Frequently encountered bites and stings encompass:

- Spider bites (e.g., redback, funnel-web, mouse, white-tailed spiders)

- Bee stings

- European wasp stings

- Scorpion stings

- Ant and centipede bites

- Mosquito bites

- Tick bites

- Snake bites

- Stings from sea creatures (like blue-ringed octopus, cone shells, box jellyfish, and stonefish)

- Bites from household pests (including fleas, bedbugs, and body lice).

Pressure bandaging and immobilization

Pressure bandaging and immobilization is useful for some bites and stings, but not all. It is recommended for:

- Snakes (Including Sea Snakes)
- Funnel-Web and Mouse Spiders
- Blue Ring Octopuses
- Cone Shells.

It is not recommended to be used for other types of bites and stings.

Pressure bandaging and immobilization are techniques used to slow the movement of venom through the lymphatic system in case of snake bites or similar emergencies. The lymphatic system is responsible for draining fluid (lymph) from body tissues back into the bloodstream.

When applying pressure bandaging, the goal is to firmly wrap the wound area to compress nearby lymph vessels. This compression helps prevent venom from spreading beyond the puncture site. If bandages are not available, makeshift items like clothing, stockings, or towels can be used.

Immobilizing the affected limb also aids in slowing venom spread by minimizing muscle movement. The lymphatic system relies on muscle contractions to propel lymph through its vessels, so immobilization can delay venom movement for several hours. These techniques are crucial initial responses to venomous bites to mitigate the effects of venom spread in the body.

Here are the steps for applying pressure bandaging and immobilization in response to a bite or sting:

> Remove any jewellery from the affected limb if possible.

> Apply a broad pressure bandage over the bite or sting site, starting from the bottom of the limb and wrapping upward. If available, mark the site with an 'X' using a pen or marker on the outermost bandage. The bandage should be firm but not overly tight. Continuously monitor the fingers or toes for changes in color, temperature, or sensation.

> Use a heavy crepe or elasticized roller bandage (10-15 centimeters wide) to apply an additional layer of bandaging. Begin just above the fingers or toes and wrap upward toward the affected limb. Ensure that the bandage does not cause numbness, tingling, or discoloration in the extremities.

> Splint the limb to minimize movement. Use sturdy objects like wood planks or magazines, securely tied or bandaged to the limb.

> Further restrict movement by tying the legs together to limit mobility.

> Keep the affected person calm and seek immediate medical assistance.

> Avoid having the person walk to the rescue vehicle; instead, bring the vehicle as close as possible to them for transport to medical help.

The old practice of using a tight tourniquet to cut off blood flow and prevent venom circulation is no longer recommended. It's important not to attempt cutting a bite to release venom or sucking out the venom from the wound. Additionally, avoid giving alcohol to the affected person to drink. These approaches lack effectiveness and could potentially exacerbate the situation.

Snake Bites

In the United States, various snake species pose potential risks, particularly during warmer months. Snakes are commonly found near wetlands, waterways, and wooded areas.

If you encounter a snake, it's important to stay calm and slowly move away from the snake to a safe distance. Some venomous snakes to be aware of in certain regions include:

- Rattlesnakes (such as the Western diamondback, Eastern diamondback, and timber rattlesnake)

- Copperheads

- Cottonmouths (also known as water moccasins)

- Coral snakes

Knowing how to identify and avoid encounters with these snakes can help minimize the risk of bites and promote safety in snake-prone regions of the United States.

Snake bite symptoms

Signs of a snake bite aren't always immediately visible, and some individuals may not feel the snake biting them at all. Symptoms may not manifest for an hour or more after the bite, making it crucial to act swiftly if a snake bite is suspected.

Depending on the type of snake involved, signs and symptoms can vary and may include:

- Immediate or delayed pain at the bite site

- Swelling, bruising, or local bleeding

- Bite marks on a limb, ranging from obvious puncture wounds to nearly invisible scratches

- Enlarged and sensitive lymph nodes located in the groin or armpit of the impacted limb.

- Faintness, dizziness

- Nausea and vomiting

- Headache

- Abdominal pain

- Blood seeping from the area where the bite occurred or from the gums.

- Double or blurred vision

- Drooping eyelids

- Difficulty speaking or swallowing

- Limb weakness or paralysis

- Difficulty breathing

- At times, there might be an initial breakdown or uncertainty, succeeded by a partial or full recovery.

First Aid for Snake Bites

➢ Follow the DRSABCD (Danger, Response, Send, Airway, Breathing, CPR, Defibrillation) protocol in case of a snake or spider bite:

➢ Call 911 and request an ambulance immediately.

➢ Lay the person down, instruct them to remain still, and provide reassurance.

➢ If possible, remove jewelry from the affected limb.

➢ Wrap a wide pressure bandage around the area where the bite occurred. Mark the location of the bite with an X on the bandage.

➢ Use an elasticized roller bandage (10–15 cm wide) starting just above the fingers or toes and wrapping upwards firmly on the limb. Ensure the bandage is tight enough that you cannot easily slide a finger underneath.

➢ Immobilize the bandaged limb using a splint.

➢ Keep the person lying down and immobile.

➢ Regularly check the color, temperature, and sensation in their fingers or toes.

➢ Record the time of the bite and when the bandage was applied. If known, mark the bite site on the skin with a pen or take a photograph. Do not wash off venom from the skin or clothing as it may aid identification.

➤ Remain by the individual's side until professional medical help arrives.

➤ Avoid having the person walk to the rescue vehicle; instead, bring the vehicle as close as possible to them.

Spider bites

The appropriate first aid response for spider bites in America depends on the species of spider and whether the spider is venomous. Common venomous spiders in America that may cause harmful bites include:

- Black widow spider

- Brown recluse spider

It's important to identify the spider if possible and seek medical attention promptly if bitten by a venomous spider. For non-venomous spider bites, basic first aid measures such as cleaning the bite area with soap and water, applying a cold compress, and taking over-the-counter pain relievers can help alleviate symptoms. If there's any concern about the bite or if symptoms worsen, it's advisable to consult a healthcare professional.

Spider bite symptoms

Common symptoms of spider bites can include:

- Intense discomfort where the bite occurred.

- Sweating

- Nausea, vomiting, and abdominal pain

- Burning sensation

- Swelling

- Blistering

First Aid for Spider Bite

➤ In the event of a spider bite, follow the DRSABCD protocol

➤ Dial 911 (or local emergency number) and request an ambulance immediately.

- Lay the person down and instruct them to remain still. Offer comfort to assist in maintaining their composure.

- Safely remove any jewelry from the affected limb.

- If the bite is on a limb, use a broad pressure bandage (10–15 cm wide) over the bite site. Mark the site with an X using a pen on the bandage.

- Wrap an elasticized roller bandage (10–15 cm wide) starting just above the fingers or toes, moving upwards on the bitten limb. Again, mark the bite site with an X on the outermost bandage. Ensure the bandage is firm but not excessively tight. Continuously monitor the color, temperature, and feeling in the fingers or toes.

- Maintain the patient in a lying down position, keeping them completely still and immobilized.

- Note the time of the bite and when the bandage was applied. If feasible, use a pen to indicate the bite area on the skin or capture it in a photo. Do not wash away venom from the skin or clothes, as it may aid in identification.

- Stay with the individual until medical assistance arrives.

- Do not attempt to make the person walk. Bring the rescue vehicle as close as possible to them for transport to medical care.

Scorpion stings

In the United States, there are different species of scorpions. Fortunately, unlike in some other parts of the world, scorpion stings in the U.S. are typically not lethal. However, certain American scorpion species can deliver a painful sting that may cause localized pain and swelling lasting several hours.

To provide first aid for scorpion stings:

- Apply a cold pack to the bite or sting area for 15 minutes. Reapply if pain persists.

- Use non-prescription pain relief medication like paracetamol.

- Change the cold pack as needed to maintain its effectiveness.

> Seek medical attention if the pain worsens or if there are any concerning symptoms.

Bee Sting

Bee stings can be sudden and alarming, especially for children playing outdoors. Knowing how to respond promptly can help alleviate panic and provide effective treatment. The first step is to remove the stinger promptly. Leaving the stinger in the skin allows more venom to be released, increasing pain and swelling.

If you are stung by a bee, wasp, or hornet, follow these steps recommended by dermatologists:

> Stay calm and walk away from the area to avoid further stings.

> Remove the stinger by scraping it off with your fingernail or a piece of gauze. Refrain from using tweezers, as they may increase the release of venom.

> Wash the sting site with soap and water to clean the area.

> Use a cold pack to reduce swelling. Seek immediate medical attention if swelling spreads to your face or neck, as this could indicate an allergic reaction.

> Watch for signs of allergic reaction such as difficulty breathing, nausea, hives, or dizziness.

> Consider using over-the-counter pain relievers like acetaminophen or ibuprofen to alleviate pain. Make sure to adhere to the dosage guidelines provided on the label at all times.

For serious reactions or multiple bee stings, prompt first aid is crucial:

> Remove the stinger as quickly as possible.
> If the person has been stung in the mouth or multiple times in a single incident (more than 10 times for adults or more than 5 times for children), seek immediate medical attention at a hospital.
> Call 911 and request an ambulance for urgent assistance.
> Administer adrenaline if it is prescribed for bee stings by the individual.

> Keep the person lying down and completely still (immobilized) until medical help arrives. This helps prevent further complications and ensures proper care upon arrival.

Wasp stings

Wasp stings are a common occurrence, especially during warmer months when people spend more time outdoors. While they can be uncomfortable, most individuals recover quickly and without complications. Wasps, similar to bees and hornets, possess a stinger used for self-defense. The stinger delivers venom—a poisonous substance—into humans during a sting.

Even without a lodged stinger, wasp venom can cause considerable pain and irritation. For individuals allergic to the venom, a serious reaction is possible. Prompt treatment is crucial in managing symptoms and preventing complications in such cases.

First aid for less severe insect stings involves several steps:

> Clean the affected area using soap and warm water.

> Use a cold compress to decrease swelling and relieve pain.

> Consider using over-the-counter pain-relieving medications and creams.

> Remain vigilant for signs of anaphylaxis (severe allergic reactions).

If you are allergic to wasp venom and have been advised by your doctor to carry self-injectable adrenaline (such as EpiPen):

> Immediately call 911 for an ambulance.

> If breathing stops, initiate resuscitation promptly.

> Follow the individual's emergency plan if one is in place.

> Administer the person's prescribed medication into the thigh.

> Apply a pressure immobilization bandage over the sting site to prevent venom spread and minimize movement.

Tick bites

Ticks are prevalent in America, acting as blood-sucking parasites. Certain species of ticks harbor disease-causing agents that pose risks to humans. Among them, the paralysis tick is notorious for its bites, which can trigger allergic reactions and, in severe cases, anaphylaxis.

Symptoms of a tick bite may manifest as:

- Rash

- Headache

- Fever

- Flu-like symptoms

- Swollen glands

- Difficulty walking

- Sensitivity to bright light

- Weakness in limbs

- Facial paralysis

It's crucial to remove the entire tick effectively. Conduct a thorough body check to ensure no ticks remain.

- Use aerosol spray containing ether to freeze and eliminate the tick. These sprays can be obtained from your pharmacy. The tick should die within about 10 minutes of applying the aerosol. Afterwards, you can brush away any remnants of the dead tick.

- For small larval ticks, apply a permethrin-containing cream to kill them before brushing them off.

- If you're unable to remove the tick using these methods, consult your doctor for assistance.

First aid for tick bites typically involves simple care, as most bites heal on their own. After removing the tick, clean the area thoroughly and apply antiseptic along with a bandage or dressing. If you encounter any of the following, it's important to seek medical help:

> Rash or swelling at the bite site
> Persistent symptoms that do not clear up
> Signs of infection or tissue damage
> Feelings of weakness, unsteadiness, or unusual sleepiness
> Double vision
> Difficulty breathing or swallowing
> Night sweats
> Fever
> Prompt medical attention is important if you notice any concerning symptoms after a tick bite.

Jellyfish Stings

Jellyfish are ocean-dwelling creatures found worldwide, characterized by soft, bell-shaped bodies and long, finger-like tentacles. These tentacles house stinging cells called nematocysts, each containing venom used for defense and capturing prey.

While jellyfish typically sting inadvertently when humans come into contact with them while swimming or walking along the beach, most stings are harmless. However, certain jellyfish stings can cause serious harm. If you or someone you're with is stung by a jellyfish and experiences life-threatening symptoms like difficulty breathing, it's essential to seek immediate medical assistance. Call 911 or head to the nearest emergency room promptly.

Certain types of jellyfish can cause serious harm due to their venomous stings. Here are some examples of jellyfish species known for their dangerous stings:

- **Box Jellyfish**: This is the most deadly jellyfish in the world, known as sea wasps. Their bodies are rectangular in shape, featuring tentacles protruding from every corner. Box jellyfish are commonly found in tropical areas, particularly along the northern coast of Australia and in the Indo-Pacific Ocean. The Australian box jellyfish is the most venomous among them.

- **Lion's Mane Jellyfish**: These are the largest jellyfish globally, growing up to more than 3 feet wide with tentacles that can reach up to 120 feet in length. Lion's mane jellyfish inhabit cooler climates, including the Arctic Ocean and the North Pacific Ocean. They are named for the mane-like appearance created by their numerous sting-covered tentacles.

- **Sea Nettle Jellyfish**: Sea nettles are large jellyfish commonly found along the Atlantic, Pacific, and Gulf coasts. They can grow over 1 foot wide and possess 24 tentacles that can extend up to 6 feet in length.

- **Portuguese Man-of-War**: Although not a true jellyfish, the Portuguese man-of-war resembles one and is known for its potent sting. These creatures inhabit tropical waters in the Atlantic, Pacific, and Indian oceans, as well as the Caribbean Sea. They have balloon-like floats to keep them afloat above water, with long tentacles and polyps extending up to about 30 feet underwater.

Symptoms

The symptoms of a jellyfish sting can vary depending on the type of jellyfish involved. For a minor jellyfish sting, you might experience slight pain, itching, burning, or throbbing sensations. The affected area may appear as a rash with red, purple, or brown patches.

However, more serious jellyfish stings can lead to severe symptoms that require immediate medical attention. These symptoms may include:

- Difficulty breathing
- Chest pain
- Muscle cramps
- Formation of skin blisters
- Numbness or tingling sensations
- Nausea or vomiting
- Difficulty swallowing (dysphagia)

- Abdominal pain
- Excessive sweating (hyperhidrosis)

Treatment for a jellyfish sting can typically be managed with first aid measures without needing to see a healthcare provider. For mild jellyfish stings, follow these steps:

➤ Rinse the affected area with seawater to wash away tentacles and venom. Avoid using freshwater, as it can activate more nematocysts.

➤ Use tweezers or wear gloves to meticulously extract any lingering tentacles from the skin.

➤ Apply vinegar or rubbing alcohol to the affected area to prevent further discharge of nematocysts. Note that vinegar should not be used for Portuguese man-of-war stings, as it may cause more venom release.

➤ To alleviate pain and reduce swelling, you can apply calamine lotion or hydrocortisone cream to the sting area. Additionally, using an ice pack or applying hot water can help relieve discomfort.

CONCLUSION

As we conclude this comprehensive guide to basic first aid, I want to express my sincere appreciation for your commitment to learning and readiness in emergency situations. Throughout these pages, we've delved into essential techniques and principles that can make a significant difference in times of crisis.

First aid is not just a skill; it's a mindset—an attitude of preparedness and compassion. By immersing yourself in the knowledge presented here, you've taken a crucial step toward becoming a confident and capable first responder. Whether you're faced with a minor injury or a life-threatening emergency, your actions can be instrumental in preserving life and promoting recovery.

The journey of learning first aid doesn't end with this book. It's an ongoing process of refining skills and staying informed about best practices. I encourage you to continue practicing the techniques discussed here and seek further training or certification if possible. Regular practice not only enhances proficiency but also builds confidence in your ability to respond effectively in challenging situations.

Remember, in moments of crisis, staying calm is key. Take a deep breath, assess the situation, and prioritize safety for yourself and those around you. Trust in your abilities and apply the knowledge you've gained with confidence.

One of the most valuable aspects of first aid is its universal applicability. Whether you're at home, in the workplace, or out in the community, the ability to provide immediate assistance can make a critical difference. Share your knowledge with others and encourage them to learn basic first aid too. Collectively, we have the capacity to establish a safer and stronger environment that benefits all. I also want to emphasize the importance of continuous learning and staying updated with advancements in first aid protocols. Medical guidelines and techniques evolve over time, so remaining informed ensures that you're equipped with the latest information and strategies to address emergent situations effectively.

As you embark on your journey as a proactive first aider, remember that your efforts contribute to the well-being of your community. By being prepared and responsive, you're making a positive impact and potentially saving lives.

In closing, I want to thank you once again for investing your time and effort into learning these vital skills. I hope this book has empowered you to take action with confidence when faced with emergencies. Stay safe, stay informed, and continue to be a beacon of support and readiness wherever you go.

Wishing you success and fulfillment in your journey as a prepared and proactive first responder.

Thank you

We want to appreciate you for taking the time to delve into "**Basic First Aid Manual Guide**." Your dedication to learning these vital techniques is truly commendable. We value your feedback and would greatly appreciate hearing your thoughts on how the book has impacted your understanding of emergency care. Your insights will help us continue to refine and improve our resources for the benefit of all.

Made in the USA
Las Vegas, NV
26 November 2024